Evidence-based Social Work

A critical stance

Mel Gray
Debbie Plath
Stephen A. Webb

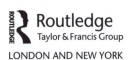

Routledge
Taylor & Francis Group

LONDON AND NEW YORK

First published 2009
by Routledge
2 Park Square, Milton Park, Abingdon, Oxon, OX14 4RN

Simultaneously published in the USA and Canada
by Routledge
270 Madison Avenue, New York, NY 10016

Routledge is an imprint of the Taylor & Francis Group, an informa business

Typeset in Times New Roman by
Pindar NZ, Auckland, New Zealand
Printed and bound in Great Britain by
TJ International Ltd, Padstow, Cornwall

British Library Cataloguing in Publication Data
A catalogue record for this book is available from the British Library

Library of Congress Cataloging-in-Publication Data
Gray, Mel, 1951–
　Evidence-based social work: a critical stance / Mel Gray, Debbie Plath,
　Stephen A. Webb.
　　p. cm.
　Includes bibliographical references and index.
　1. Evidence-based soical work. 2. Social service—Practice. I. Plath,
Debbie. II. Webb, Stephen A., 1956- III. Title.
　HV10.5.G73 2009
　361.3'2—dc22　　　　　　　　　　　2008050970

ISBN10: 0-415-46822-1 (hbk)
ISBN10: 0-415-46823-X (pbk)
ISBN10: 0-203-87662-8 (ebk)

ISBN13: 978-0-415-46822-0 (hbk)
ISBN13: 978-0-415-46823-7 (pbk)
ISBN13: 978-0-203-87662-6 (ebk)

Evidence-based Social Work

Evidence-based practice (EBP) is now a core element of many governments' approaches to policy-making and social intervention. It has become a powerful movement that promises to change the content and structure of social work and its allied professions. Its emergence has generated much debate and raised challenging questions, however, particularly at the interface of research, policy and practice.

This book provides a critical analysis of evidence-based practice in social work. It introduces readers to the fast-changing research, policy, legislative and practice contexts. It discusses what constitutes knowledge in social work, the values and beliefs that lie behind evidence-based practice, and the problems of implementation, formalization and resource management. Reflecting on the challenges of transferring evidence-based practice to frontline social work practice, Gray, Plath and Webb argue that social work practice is not easily measured and systematized into best practice guidelines that disseminate proven diagnostic and effective intervention knowledge.

Using actor network theory for the first time in the social work literature, *Evidence-based Social Work* illuminates how adopting the methodology and language of evidence-based practice fundamentally alters the conditions under which social work takes place. This book is vital reading for academics, practitioners and students with an interest in contemporary social work practice and research.

Mel Gray is Professor of Social Work and a full-time researcher in the Institute for Social Well-being at the University of Newcastle, Australia.

Debbie Plath is Senior Lecturer in Social Work in the School of Humanities and Social Science at the University of Newcastle, Australia.

Stephen A. Webb is Professor of Human Sciences and Director of the Institute for Social Well-being at the University of Newcastle, Australia.

To Dave, Greg and Penni
and in loving memory of Mary and Philip Webb

Contents

x   *Contents*

Illustrations

Figures

Tables

Acknowledgements

Evidence-based practice is a subject fraught with controversy within social work circles but the debates it engenders are enriching and worthwhile for the profession, which prides itself on its value-driven, ethical practice. In undertaking this research we have debated the complex issues among ourselves and sought advice from colleagues and eminent researchers in the field. And certain people have been an invaluable catalyst and support along the way. We would especially like to thank all those who so willingly responded to our requests for information and clarification and would like to mention in particular Haluk Soydan, Bruce Thyer, Aron Shlonsky, Joel Fischer, David Stoesz, Riaan van Zyl, Eileen Gambrill, Joan Zlotnick, Robert Boruch, Edgar Marthinsen, Terje Ogden, Keiji Akiyama and Stan Witkin. They, along with many others cited in this book, have made an invaluable contribution to contemporary ideas about evidence-based social work and its workability or otherwise. Even its staunchest advocates are seriously grappling with issues of translation and implementation and how to increase the uptake of evidence-based social work by human service agencies, including managers and practitioners. An area that we have not explored but which comes to mind as one meriting future attention is that of the service user as a target for education about evidence-based practice. Perhaps if service users were better informed, they might demand that their social workers use this approach! Such is the nature of evidence-based practice that there is much still to debate before we can seriously advocate it as the model of choice in social work practice.

We are all extremely grateful to our partners and families for their whole-hearted support and encouragement. Mel thanks Dave, Debra-Ann and Barry Jon, who have been behind her and are integral to everything she does.

Debbie is grateful to Mel and Stephen for providing the opportunity to participate in this project and to Greg, Thomas and Aidan for putting up with it while she did.

Stephen warmly thanks Penni for her patience, kindness and love without which, as ever, this work would not have been possible. Her continuing personal support and selflessness is steadfast and always encouraging of intellectual endeavour.

Finally, of course, this is a Routledge book and we are extremely grateful to Grace McInnes, our commissioning editor. It was Grace's idea to embark on the project and we thank her for her patience, support and encouragement throughout.

We would also like to thank Eloise Cook, who worked closely with us until she moved to a different position at Routledge in October 2008 and Khanam Virjee who took us across the finishing line.

Introduction

Evidence-based thinking has come to underpin the approaches of many governments to policy-making and social intervention, and has become part of the
machinery of audit and governance over the past decade. It has far-reaching
international and national significance. Evidence as a systematic approach to policy
and practice formation has influenced a wide range of disciplines – including
medicine, public management, education, developmental studies, criminology
and social work – with the intention of increasing transparency by the use of
rigorous, standardized and up-to-date evaluations. Perhaps, as an indication of
the very significant impact of evidence-based approaches, the US case of the
'No Child Left Behind' Act of 2001 offers useful illustration. It is the most
wide-ranging piece of public legislation since Johnson's 'Great Society' Act of
1965 and features evidence as the central methodological platform for reform,
mentioning 'scientifically-based research' 111 times in the text. It appears that the
grand narrative of science is unashamedly reborn in the midst of the postmodern
'anything goes' narrative and the 'anti-science' onslaught of critical theory. In the
UK, evidence-based practice has been championed by government ministers as part
of their benchmarking and modernizing strategy in all areas of the public sector.
The evidence-based success story is widely felt, with some claiming, for example,
that it has become the cornerstone of UK health policy (Trinder and Reynolds
2000). The influence of evidence-based practice in social work has steadily
increased over the past few years, although the emergence of such practice has not
been without its critics. As an area of contestation, it has generated much debate
and raised many challenging questions, particularly at the interface of research,
policy and practice in social work. There are undoubtedly many competing ideas
about evidence-based approaches and different models from which one can
learn a great deal. The competing ideas are complex and involve not only highly
technical problems of logic and scientific axioms, but also larger epistemological
considerations about interpretation, decision-making and the status of knowledge.
While some of these fall within the narrow range of scientific methodology, others
have provoked philosophical questions about the nature of truth and knowledge,
and about distinctions between fact and value. These debates are embedded in
historic assumptions about the nature of reality and how it can best be understood.
At a more practical level, advances in the evidence-based agenda have raised

important issues about the professional status, legitimacy, autonomy and authority of social work.

This book provides a comprehensive analysis of evidence-based practice in social work, focusing on current advances in the field, as we map contemporary developments in epistemology, methodology and practice interventions for social work and identify the key components that constitute various strands of thinking. In undertaking this analysis, we draw on the considerable empirical insights and theoretical research of actor network theory (Callon and Law 1982; Callon 1986; Latour 1987, 1988; Law 1999).[1] An actor is seen not just as a 'point object' but rather as an association of heterogeneous elements, themselves constituting a network. Each actor is thus itself also a simplified network (Law 1992). In actor network theory, interactions and associations between actors and networks are the important thing, and actors are seen only as the sum of their interactions with other actors and networks.

The book tells the story of evidence-based practice as it unfolds and has come to be realized in shaping new agendas, networks and priorities for social work. We contrast, for instance, the investment that has been made in systematic knowledge reviews as guidelines for best practice, over say the development of evidence-based protocols to directly inform decision-making. It is shown how the use of best practice guidelines to disseminate proven knowledge of effective interventions has tended to predominate. It is our contention that these developments are best understood in terms of their *situatedness* and complex research, policy and organizational *context*. Thus we demonstrate how social work has been affected by the production, transmission and reception of evidence-based practice. In doing this, we identify both the restricted and broad sense to which the concept of evidence-based practice has been deployed. We contend that the broad sense in which it is used is such as to make it almost meaningless at the level of frontline practice, while the narrower conception is more idiosyncratic and has various advantages and disadvantages for social work. As Webb (2006) has shown, the emergence of 'technologies of care', such as risk management and evidence-based practice, take place in a specific environment that lends itself to the hardening of certain strategies, interventions and processes. They are rational responses to the nature of changing social forms in a risk-dominated organizational culture. Social work is increasingly rendered into a technical calculable form. Evidence-based practice comprises networks that reframe objectivity through the accomplishment of dynamic operating systems (Webb 2006: 142–143).

Throughout the book it is maintained that demonstrating a *critical stance* in relation to evidence-based practice is crucial for social work at both the policy and frontline practice levels. Very much in keeping with traditions of learning in social work, the 'critical stance' refers to a particular manner in which practitioners, students and teachers engage within the practice environment. Thus the critical stance is an attitude or disposition towards oneself, others and the object of inquiry that challenges and impels social workers to reflect, understand and act in a milieu of potentiality. This means that policy-makers, practitioners and students should have a critical awareness of the values, ethics and beliefs that underlie both the formalization of evidence-based practice *as well as* issues that relate to implementation and outcomes. Moreover, the ambiguity, complexity and contradictions inherent in much of social work suggest the necessity of adopting a critical stance for practice. At a substantive level, we use Ferguson's (2003) concept of 'critical-best practice' to analyze the interplay between a critically reflexive stance and evidence-based methodologies and to draw out the implications for practice.

It is our contention that the case for or against evidence-based social work needs to be argued rather than assumed. It needs to be critically examined rather than asserted. At the present time, the case for the deployment of evidence-based practice in social work cannot meet evidence-based practice's own internal criteria for the admissibility of research. We concur with the editors of the *British Educational Research Journal* who, in the editorial 'Old whine in new battles' (Stronach and Hustler 2001: 524), critically considered the possible influx of evidence-based strategies in the field of education in concluding that 'there is no substantial evidence to vindicate its application or to justify "transfer" arguments from medical or health studies'. As conceived in terms of evidence-based social work, the program of evidence-based practice cannot meet its own criteria of rigour or validity except retrospectively. However, we also agree that the emergence of evidence-based practice offers an opportunity to investigate why, in some quarters of social work, there are advocates who might wish to endorse this program and explore what this tells us about the status, role and changing nature of social work. In other words, the advent of evidence-based practice is as much an argument for a creative exploration and offers an opportunity to take a critical stance in developing arguments against certain variants of evidence-based practice.

In the concluding chapter, we show that, at present, there is no explicit 'framework for practice' but rather a *policy formation* and *research programming* agenda for evidence-based practice. In plain terms, frontline practitioners currently have a limited sense of what evidence-based practice actually is, let alone how to implement it. Indeed, the slowness with which evidence-based practice is being adopted in social work has lessons both for further work on evidence-based practice itself and also for future implementation of innovations intended to improve social care. However, the adoption of both the methodology and language of evidence-based practice, as the basis for a comprehensive policy program, means that it will fundamentally alter the conditions under which social work takes place and the working relationship with service users. Evidence-based practice has become a powerful movement that promises to change the content and structure of social work and its allied professions. Indications of its impact are discussed with reference to new organizations, such as the Social Care Institute for Excellence and the Campbell Collaboration, as well as journals, such as *Evidence-based Mental Health, Evidence and Policy, Research Evaluation* and *Research on Social Work Practice.*

The primary audience for the book is social work students, at undergraduate, postgraduate and post-qualifying levels, social work educators and practitioners, as well as social and healthcare managers and organizational administrators and policy-makers charged with providing evidence of effectiveness in resource allocation and use. It is intended as a primary text for undergraduate, masters and doctoral courses in social work. Not only will it introduce students to contemporary issues and debates surrounding evidence-based policy and practice, it will also assist them to engage in and advance these debates in the interests of critical best practice. It will help practitioners, managers and administrators to gain a deeper insight into the machinations of the workplace and the impact of evidence-led policies and processes, again so that they might contribute to the smooth functioning of their organizations in the best interests of service users. In short, understanding evidence-led policy and practice enhances accountability. The book should also be of interest to other occupations and professions involved in social and healthcare or in the human services broadly defined.

Many social work programs have a course entitled 'Evidence-based practice' and, given the contemporary practice environment, not having such a course in a social work education program would be very much an oversight. This book constitutes an ideal text on which to base a course on evidence-based practice. It is also relevant to courses on:

1 social work theory, method and knowledge development, including debates on what counts as knowledge and what exactly evidence-based intervention is;
2 social work practice, especially skills in decision-making;
3 social work research methods, especially its epistemological foundations and research design aspects;
4 social work undergraduate and postgraduate thesis work.

It covers the full range of contemporary thinking on evidence-based practice. Chapter 1 examines the emergence of evidence-based practice and proposes that evidence-based social work entails the mobilization of a specialist research infrastructure to guide particular approaches to practice. We consider how evidence-based social work has been shaped by the historical association that the profession has had with research and also by the current research, political, legislative and organizational contexts in which social work is practised. Some of the key concepts of concern in the book are introduced and delineated, including 'evidence', 'evidence-based practice', 'evidence-based social work' and 'evidence-based knowledge', and some of the myths surrounding these concepts are exposed. We show that there are important distinctions to be drawn between 'knowledge', 'evidence' and 'information'. The process of knowledge formalization is examined in Chapter 1 as a way of understanding how practice is negotiated at individual, organizational and policy levels in social work.

Chapter 2 offers a detailed account of a particular stance on evidence-based practice that has come to dominate language and thinking on the topic, i.e., the scientific–experimental–behaviourist approach associated with 'gold standard' evidence. We consider the inadequacies of the approach in conceptual, methodological and practical terms. This explanation and analysis, together with case examples from the Cochrane Collaboration, offer resources for the social work practitioner engaged in designing, using or critiquing experimental research and systematic reviews as a source of evidence for practice. Chapter 2 is designed to assist the practitioner to understand both the strengths and limitations of such research and to appreciate the perspective of the advocates of experimental design. For those social workers who feel alienated by the language of experimental studies and randomized controlled trials, we have tried to demystify these research designs.

Having critically examined the dominant view on evidence-based practice, we then pose in Chapter 3 the question of whether there is a particular social work approach to such practice. We explore this question by locating evidence-based practice within the traditions of social work theories, ethics and practice principles. Chapter 3 offers the practitioner, faced with confusing or conflicting views on evidence, a framework for understanding various perspectives on evidence-based practice. We tease out the different values, goals and processes that influence positivist, pragmatic, political and postmodern discourses on evidence-based practice in social work. Chapter 3 provides social workers with a way of making sense of the debates and tensions that have surrounded the emergence of evidence-based social work, suggesting that there is a way forward for social work in integrating these different approaches to suit the context and presenting issues. We have argued that evidence-based social work is an amalgam of scientific–positivist and interpretivist–practical and political considerations.

Building on the premise that context, presenting issues and key players all work to shape evidence-based social work approaches in different settings, Chapter 4 describes how evidence-based social work has been translated into different international contexts. Diffusion and actor network theory are used as frameworks for examining the global spread of evidence-based practice, beginning with its development in the USA and continuing with its translation to international contexts in Europe, the Asia–Pacific region, Israel and Canada. Key actors and organizational networks that have facilitated local translations of evidence-based social work in these countries are identified. While invariably there are local distinctions, a list of commonalities of evidence-based social work across these contexts is also delineated.

Chapter 5 further develops the diffusion analysis of Chapter 4 by providing some detailed observations on the development of evidence-based social work in the UK, through the lens of actor network theory. We use the UK case example to describe how diffusion occurs within a specific context by focusing on the social work research, policy and professional communities which are the networks of institutions that give voice to particular discourses in social work. Looking beyond evidence-based social work as decision-making by individual practitioners, we examine the processes, actors and networks that have facilitated the formalization and implementation of evidence-based social work in the UK. The tension between 'soft' and 'hard' approaches to evidence-based social work has been a feature of the UK situation as networks respond to different audiences and critics.

In Chapter 6 we examine the formal and informal aspects, both social and technical, that impact on the implementation of evidence-based practice for social work. We propose that the future of evidence-based social work depends on the ways in which key stakeholders – policy-makers, funding bodies, managers, decision-makers and professional leaders – deal with researchers and frontline practitioners, particularly in situations of resistance. The macro and micro factors that work against the implementation of evidence-based social work are identified, along with strategies to address them. These strategies recognize the limitation of placing the onus of implementation on the individual practitioner when, as we argue, knowledge translation involves the mobilization of research systems to support practice. Evidence-based social work is regarded as a dynamic and imperfect process that involves research, policy and practice infrastructure pushing the practitioner in a particular direction.

The practitioner experience of evidence-based social work is the focus of Chapter 7, where we draw together the themes and issues identified throughout the book by relating these to several specific social work practice scenarios and to some of the current issues encountered by social workers in practice. We explain how a critical understanding of evidence-based social work can aid the practitioner in negotiating practice contexts. As systems are mobilized to implement evidence-based social work, it is the integrity of key players that will influence the degree to which improving the quality of life of vulnerable and powerless people is upheld as the central concern. This remains the real challenge of evidence-based social work.

Note

1 Methodologically, actor network theory has two major approaches: one is to 'follow the actor', via interviews and ethnographic research; the other is to examine inscriptions. Inscriptions – including texts and images of many sorts, databases, and the like – are central to knowledge work. Some (e.g., Callon *et al*. 1986; Latour and Woolgar 1991) say that texts (including journal articles, conference papers and presentations, grant proposals, and patents) are among the major, if not *the* major, products of scientific work. Inscriptions make action at a distance possible by stabilizing work in such a way that it can travel across space and time and be combined with other work.

1 New horizons in evidence

Over the past decade, evidence-based practice has been hailed as signalling a new era of progress and offering great promise for social work. For some, however, it is the ghost in the machine because it carries with it a propensity for detrimental effects, which savagely undercuts core principles, values and traditional ways of working in social work. As a recent innovation, it has also heralded significant change that will move social work into unknown territories. This opening chapter begins our critical exploration of the emergence, parameters, consequences, ambitions and ideologies of evidence-based practice as it is seen to impact on social work. Trinder (2000) proclaimed the emergence of evidence-based practice as one of the success stories of the 1990s. But was she right? As a methodological program, based on a particular epistemology, it certainly came to dominate medicine towards the end of the last decade of the twentieth century. However, it only really began to influence social work in the late 1990s. Given its roots in evidence-based medicine, it is not surprising that it has been most successful in those disciplines closest to medicine but only partially successful in disciplines like social work. For us, evidence-based practice is an emergent phenomenon that has yet to be fully realized as 'evidence-based social work'. We suggest that evidence-based social work is best defined as entailing the mobilization of a specialist research infrastructure that can guide particular interventions, support best practice governance and demonstrate positive outcomes for service users. Evidence-based practice *becomes* evidence-based social work at the point when it materializes, is performed and made durable in a more or less fixed set of locations within social work, e.g., in social work agencies or cultures of social work practice. The emphasis is on the transportability of evidence-based practice *into* social work based on a series of implementation moves to become 'evidence-based social work'. As we show, there is a need for micro studies of methodological and policy formation, particularly around the challenging issues of implementation in social work. Such studies would allow us to understand how processes of improvization, purification and channelling are translated into local and national contexts, giving insights into the embedding – or not – of evidence-based methodology in day-to-day social work practice. In this regard, this chapter advances some of the key arguments of the book that turn on the following statements:

1   Evidence-based practice is essentially a process of formalization driven by evidence-based policy which allies with attempts to legislate a particular definition of 'scientific inquiry' (Maxwell 2004: 36) and, in some forms, a return to experimental design studies involving large, randomized samples recreated on the clinical model with its many attendant weaknesses (see Chapter 2).

2   Evidence-based practice is very different from the empirical clinical practice, effectiveness and practice evaluation models in social work that developed in the UK and USA respectively and the more recent, empirically supported interventions model.

3   Strictly speaking, evidence-based practice rests on the accumulation of evidence over time studied systematically through knowledge reviews of empirical research or, in its purist 'gold standard' sense, meta-analysis of experimental randomized controlled trial studies. Importantly, 'evidence' derives from multiple research studies over time and not from the application of the findings of particular studies in single instances of policy or practice. In its translation to social work, as an approach to practice, there has been a heavy focus on individual practitioners locating the 'best available evidence', which might include a range of research methodologies.

4   However, we argue that evidence-based practice is not simply about how individual practitioners locate and use evidence in practice, or how they integrate research and practice, or even how they make judgements and decisions and whether or not they use empirical evidence to inform everyday decisions about interventions. It is much more complex than this. It involves, for example, the establishment of regulatory orientations, formal networks, organizational systems, standardized practice cultures, best practice guidelines, knowledge reviews, and models of implementation based on accumulated evidence over time. It often involves intermediary – professional – bodies conducting systematic reviews and developing protocols and guidelines to make it easier for practitioners to apply the best available evidence to practice.

5   Current articulations and developments around evidence-based social work are not grounded in a coherent or programmatic theory and there is a great deal of contestability about what constitutes evidence-based practice, what counts as knowledge and how we should define it. As such, the case for or against evidence-based social work needs to be argued for rather than merely assumed.

Despite the proclivity in social work for empirical investigation, beginning with scientific charity or philanthropy in the late 1890s, one might expect that concerns with science-based practice would have created fertile ground for the flourishing of evidence-based social work. But this has not been the case and studies examining the use of research to inform practice since the 1970s to the present day have consistently shown that the uptake of research by social workers is low and sporadic (Corcoran 2007; Gambrill 2006b; Mullen and Bacon 2004; Mullen, Bellamy *et al.* 2005). Hence Corcoran (2007: 548) concluded that there remains 'a stuttering delay between the findings from science and their application in everyday, routine [social work] practice'. But evidence-based practice is not simply about how social workers use evidence to inform everyday decisions (see also Gambrill 2006a, 2006b). It is crucially part of a regimen that authorizes and standardizes not only the types of practice intervention that are permissible and those which are not, but also the types of research that are admissible as evidence. Thus we shall see how an evidence-based intervention is not merely the 'decision act' but is linked to a complex array of socio-technical background factors derived from a 'networked evidence system' without which evidence-based practice cannot flourish. Gambrill (in Thyer and Kazi 2004: 215) recognizes the importance of these networks and highlights the role of professional, accrediting and licensing organizations, professional schools of social work, agency managers and personnel, frontline practitioners, citizens and service users, including advocacy groups, and politicians and legislators, who influence the funding of programs in evidence-based practice, not to mention research organizations and centres generating systematic reviews, like the Cochrane and Campbell Collaborations. In analyzing these complex formalization pathways, evidence-based practice in social work is thus best characterized as an emerging actor network, i.e., 'an association of different elements that hold together for some common purpose' (McCarthy and Martin-McDonald 2007: 84), such that resources become 'concentrated in a few places ... which are connected with one another – the links and the mesh ... [and] transform the scattered resources into a net that may seem to extend everywhere' (Latour 1987: 180).

In later chapters, we show how actor network theory enables us to understand how this macro-level 'mesh' gives the impression that evidence-based practice has a wide reach when, in reality, it has had little impact on the day-to-day practice of social work. To be successful, 'networks of aligned interests [have to be] ... created through the enrolment of a sufficient body of allies and the translation of their interests so that they are willing to participate in particular ways of thinking and acting that maintain the network' (Walsham and Sahay 1999: 42).

We will demonstrate that social work is still a long way from achieving this form of cohesive network. While it has produced key actors who have vigorously promoted evidence-based practice within social work, they have not yet succeeded in enrolling practitioners to translate this approach into daily practice with service users. Through actor network analysis, we study the way in which evidence-based practice has been transported into social work. But before we get to this, we examine some key concepts used in evidence-based practice in this opening chapter, the research methodology it promotes (Chapter 2) and a framework for analyzing evidence-based social work (Chapter 3).

It is our contention that a proper appreciation of what constitutes evidence-based practice and how it comes to be constructed must necessarily take account of the fast-changing nature not only of social work but also of the research, policy, legislative and organizational contexts in which it is practised. We pose critical questions about how and why social work is receptive – or not – to the emerging evidence-based practice agenda and its consequent variable and uneven impact on social work. We begin by examining the key concepts we use in talking about evidence-based practice.

Introducing the key concepts

Evidence

In its general usage, 'evidence' means proven or undisputed facts. However, we know that discerning the facts, or deciding what is true, is no easy matter. Still, when considering the notion of evidence, it is wise to bear in mind that it has something to do with determining the facts or deciding what counts as truth. More specifically, it has to do with how we come to determine the facts in particular situations. When it comes to evidence-based practice, a crucial issue is the method we use to determine what counts as evidence. Advocates of evidence-based practice argue that the most reliable grounds on which to base practice are those which derive from empirical or scientific research. For this reason, there is some confusion in the social work literature between the terms 'evidence' and 'empirical', since the latter was used in the early US notion of 'empirically based practice' (Jayaratne and Levy 1979). However, as we shall see in Chapter 4, evidence-based practice is not an extension of the empirical clinical practice model but represents a new approach to social work practice which derives from evidence-based medicine. Nevertheless, the earlier empirically based practice and more recent evidence-based practice approach share a commitment to the 'scientific' method as the best way of determining reliable knowledge on which to base practice.

The earlier, empirically based practice model – and the researcher–practitioner model which preceded it, discussed more fully in Chapter 4 – were interested in demonstrating that social work intervention was effective, and, once it had been proven that certain interventions were effective with particular problems, these should be applied routinely in those situations. Hence this became known as the 'effectiveness movement' in the USA. In the UK, it was expressed in the notion of 'practice evaluation', which was a major precursor to evidence-based practice, as we shall see in Chapter 5. Thus evidence has become tied to 'what works' in practice. But this is a misleading reduction of the meaning of evidence within evidence-based practice remembering that we have already established that it is intimately tied to beliefs about legitimate grounds on which to base practice. In its translation to social work, there are wide-ranging views on what counts as legitimate knowledge, which some have placed on an 'evidence continuum' (see Barber, in White 2008 and McNeece and Thyer 2004; Figure 1.2). Those who take a narrow view argue for knowledge which derives from experimental or 'gold standard' research, i.e., research which employs randomized controlled trials. Those who take a broader view argue that more than scientific data constitutes knowledge for practice. In fact, scientific data are of no use whatsoever until they are translated into usable information and a complex network of factors determines the usability and relevance of information for practitioners. A related issue is whether or not practitioners will seek to draw on research and apply it to their practice. Producing evidence does not lead automatically to evidence-based social work. So, as we shall see, a social worker who claims that she is using the 'best available evidence' to inform her practice is not necessarily an 'evidence-based social worker', even if she is basing her decisions on evidence-based protocols. It is really important to realize that evidence-based practice is not just about using evidence in decision-making but is a systematic approach to practice which follows a number of steps in which practitioners formulate an answerable question, locate the evidence to answer this question, critically appraise the evidence, taking into account the practitioner's expertise and the patient's values and circumstances, and evaluate the effectiveness and efficiency of these steps in the evidence-based practice process (see Chapter 2).

Proponents of evidence-based practice believe that social workers ignore research evidence at their peril (Gambrill 2006a, 2006b). In their critiques of evidence-based practice, opponents, however, point to the miniscule role that strictly defined evidence, as promulgated by the narrowly conceived evidence-based practice program, can and does play in frontline practice. There are more important factors, they argue, not least the relationship of trust between client or patient and practitioner, people's desire for personal medical services, the context of practice, the personality of the patient, the severity of the problem, and so on (Charlton 1997).

As we shall see in this book, those who oppose the strict, narrow, scientific view of evidence argue that there are many sources and forms of evidence relating to realistic, non-scientific factors, such as practitioner experience, expertise and judgement; available resources and the way in which they are distributed; and prevailing values, ideologies, habits and traditions. This broader view of evidence that characterizes social work considerations about the effectiveness of research or practice evaluation (Davies, in Gambrill 2006b) is very different from that implied in *evidence-based practice*. In fact, there is a huge difference between evaluation and other types of evidence. In many definitions of research, as well as Institutional Review Board (IRB) protocols in the USA, practice evaluation is excluded. Thus it is important to understand that the core values, processes and methodologies of evidence-based practice are very different from evaluation and other forms of research, such as action and intervention research (see Hammersley 2003). In the USA, where the Society for Social Work and Research (SSWR) has strongly promoted evidence-based social work, though others are now joining forces, as we show in Chapter 4, debate continues as to the equation of evidence with knowledge produced by randomized controlled trials as the 'gold standard' of evidence-based practice. Here, and in many social work circles, the emphasis is on finding the 'best *available* evidence' and there is some, though not unanimous, agreement that sometimes the best evidence might come from qualitative research studies. But, as we shall see in Chapter 2, in the strict evidence-based practice program 'evidence' means scientific facts supported and accumulated from multiple experimental studies over time. It is reached through a rigorous review methodology known as systematic review (SR), which may or may not include meta-synthesis – the application of statistical tests to results across randomized controlled trial studies –also sometimes referred to as 'knowledge reviews'. They are not the same as conventional literature reviews, which review all – or at least as much as possible – of the available literature on a given topic. Systematic reviews only include reviews of empirical studies deemed to be of high methodological rigour and quality – with randomized controlled trials[1] (RCTs) being the highest quality available. That is, high methodological rigour accrues from multiple studies, employing a specific methodology, which confirm prior findings. Hence an important part of the methodology of systematic reviews, and meta-synthesis, relates to decisions about the quality of the research to be included, based on the criteria of objectivity, rigour, reliability and validity. In conclusion, if we want a quick definition of 'evidence', then it is a cumulative body of knowledge developed over time through empirical research.

Evidence-based practice

Evidence-based practice began in medicine in the early 1990s. Its primary source is Sackett *et al.*'s (1997, 2000) *Evidence-based Medicine: how to practice and teach EBM* and the latest edition revised by Strauss *et al.* (2005). Thyer (2008a) notes that those who wish to discuss evidence-based practice intelligently should be familiar with these primary sources. We have noted that this is not the same as practice evaluation or effectiveness research or empirically based practice. Gambrill (in Thyer and Kazi 2004: 217), too, emphasizes that evidence-based practice is not an extension of these prior research-for-practice initiatives:

> Evidence-based practice differs in a number of ways from empirical social work practice as this is described in published sources, including the rigour and completeness of research reviews, avoidance of inflated claims of effectiveness, and attention to ethical issues such as informed choice. It also differs from the practice guidelines movement in the comprehensiveness of its approach to enhancing quality of services and attention to ethical issues, helping staff to acquire critical appraisal skills, and avoiding inflated claims regarding effectiveness.

Having established what evidence-based practice is not, let us briefly examine some major themes about what it is from within the social work and wider literature.

Evidence-based practice as an alternative to authority-based practice

As we have seen, evidence-based practice is said to be clearly distinguishable from earlier research-for-practice initiatives in social work, in that it 'draws on the results of systematic, rigorous, critical appraisal of research related to important practice questions ... evidence-based practice requires helpers to search for evidence and share what is found' (Gambrill, in Thyer and Kazi 2004: 216). Corcoran and Vandiver (in Roberts and Yeager 2006: 59) present evidence-based practice as 'a process of utilizing a variety of databases to find an appropriate guide to an intervention for a particular diagnostic condition'. This requires that practitioners inform clients about current research relating to their problem and interventions available to deal with it. The evidence-based practice approach requires the integration of the best research evidence available with the practitioner's clinical expertise and the patient's unique values and circumstances (Strauss *et al*. 2005: 1), i.e., it takes the client's preferences into account in the belief that they are in a position to make informed choices based on the information given to them by the practitioner. For Soydan (2007: 317), 'the golden rule of evidence-based practice is to create transparency and open communication with the client and other stakeholders related to the client'. Gambrill (1999, 2001, 2006a, 2006b), too, highlights the importance of transparency in preventing authority-based professional practice in terms of which practitioners rely more heavily on their expertise. Transparency is said to be enhanced by client involvement, by informing clients about the 'quality' of available evidence, the degree of existing knowledge about a problem, and the effectiveness of the intervention being suggested by the practitioner – but there is, as yet, no evidence of this occurring in practice.

One important line of justification for evidence-based practice is that it subjects professional authority to public scrutiny. Evidence-based practice requires that practitioners make their uncertainties explicit by placing in the public domain the information on which they draw. In theory, evidence-based practice requires that practitioners inform clients when no scientifically tested treatments are available. Since admitting 'I don't know' and owning up to mistakes is important in evidence-based practice (Gambrill 2006b), the practice is also presented as a process of professional learning. Evidence-based practice generates tools for learning – relating to 'how to' ask the right questions, 'how to' critically appraise evidence, 'how to' make clinical decisions and so on – and generates clinical practice guidelines for practitioners. This means that practitioners need appraisal skills, not only to appraise the 'best research evidence' available but also to detect non-evidence-based clinical guidelines, such as those devised by managers and other authority-based sources. As stated by Gambrill (in Thyer and Kazi 2004: 223):

> Negative consequences of premature diffusion of 'practice guidelines' (not based on sound evidence) include formalising unsound practices, reducing practice variations they may standardise to 'average' rather than best practice, inhibiting innovation, preventing individual clients from being dealt with discreetly and sensitively, and producing undesirable shifts in the balance of power between different professional groups; for example, between clinicians and academics.

Note the language Gambrill uses: formalizing evidence, standardizing best practice. She consistently emphasizes that more than 'clinical expertise' is required and clearly wishes to take a more holistic approach to evidence-based social work than that narrowly defined in medicine. However, while prescriptions for transparency, accountability, attention to ethical issues, and service-user involvement are laudable aspirations, there is little research to show that these are actually occurring at the level of frontline practice and Gambrill acknowledges this. We have also been unable to identify any concrete instances of a client's being involved in an evidence-based decision or intervention pathway. While Gambrill's contributions are warmly persuasive, Webb (2006: 159) has criticized her for deploying rhetorical devices in her defence of evidence-based practice and in effectively creating a panacea of all admissible parts in its definition as a means of forestalling potential dissent. He claims that she defines 'evidence-based social work' so broadly that it becomes a catch-all phrase for much of what social work already is, but adds to this an emphasis on the new managerial culture of transparency and accountability. What Gambrill is actually doing with her conception of evidence-based social work is to try to stabilize interpretations of what counts, such that it resembles an absolute definition with fixed but loose reference points. With her perspective, the evidence-based project necessarily gets more complicated because she needs to reinscribe in it what threatens to interrupt its course – values, service user perspectives and transparency. But the cascade of Gambrill's translation, while maintaining safety, abandons the principle of rigour and validity so prized by the purists (e.g., Thyer) and thus ceases to authorize it. Either the principle of rigour and validity has to be scrapped, or else with Gambrill it has to be reinscribed to incorporate catch-all phrases. The problem, as we see it, with Gambrill's perspective on evidence-based social work is that she never really considers frontline practitioners or their techniques of practice. She considers only a set of social work competences that are shuffled around to accommodate her reinscribed evidence-based agenda.

Evidence-based practice as a practice framework

Within social work, evidence-based practice is seen as a practice framework which rests on the belief that better outcomes for clients ensue from direct practice, policy, management and administration based on empirical knowledge rather than on, among other things, tradition, professional authority, practice wisdom or commonsense (Gambrill 2006b; Mullen *et al.* 2008; Thyer, in Roberts and Yeager 2006). It is largely seen as 'a *way of doing practice*, a way of assessing, intervening, and evaluating based on a set of assumptions and values' (Mullen *et al.* 2008: 2 emphasis added; see also Roberts and Yeager 2006: 24) so as to bring research and practice closer together. Or, as Gambrill (2006b) notes, it is a way of closing the gap between research and practice. The aim is to 'strengthen the scientific knowledge base supporting ... *intervention*' (Soydan 2007: 2 emphasis added), the pivot around which social work turns. This is sometimes referred to as the interventionist approach to evidence and is reflected in developments that have taken place at the University of Oxford, with the establishment of the Centre for Evidence-based Intervention (see Chapter 5). Here the bridge between practice and research is sought by utilizing the evaluation of behavioural interventions for psychosocial problems and in combining a matrix of randomized trials, systematic reviews and other evaluation designs. The interventions involve specifying a target population that treatments will assist, testing the intervention and comparing with groups that do not receive the intervention. In this view, it is not dissimilar from the empirically supported interventions approach emanating from the American Psychological Association (APA), discussed in Chapter 4.

Evidence-based practice as a guide to decision-making

A third way in which evidence-based practice is presented in social work is as a guide to decision-making. For example, McCracken and Marsh (2008: 301) refer to evidence-based practice as a 'process of using research findings to aid clinical decision making'. Mullen *et al.* (2007) refer to empirically supported interventions (ESIs), mentioned above, as relating to the micro process of determining the relevance of particular interventions to specific client conditions, circumstances and preferences within the wider macro process of evidence-based practice, that is, the broader process of finding empirical evidence that supports the effectiveness and efficiency of various assessment and intervention options. Mullen *et al.* (2007: 1) highlight that, within this micro process of decision-making, practitioner expertise *is* important. Since 'the research on human information processing, perception, and problem solving ... rel[ies] heavily on judgmental heuristics or rules of thumb', reflection and critical thinking are required: 'evidence-based practice pushes the practitioner to improve the quality of decisions made by systematically reviewing information from rigorous data-gathering efforts instead of relying on customary practice or agency policy' (McCracken and Marsh 2008: 301). Thus McCracken and Marsh (2008) emphasize the importance of evidence and practitioner expertise in evidence-based practice decision-making. But, as shall be seen, we argue that it is much broader than this.

Evidence-based social work

One definition of evidence-based social work that is offered emphasizes the necessity of predictable results for intervention outcomes and empirically verified actions:

> Evidence-based [social work] dictates that professional judgments and behavior should be guided by two distinct but interdependent principles. First, whenever possible, practice should be grounded on prior findings that demonstrate empirically that certain actions performed with a particular type of client or client system are likely to produce predictable, beneficial, and effective results .... Secondly, every client system, over time, should be individually evaluated to determine the extent to which the predicted results have been attained as a direct consequence of the practitioner's actions.
>
> (Cournoyer and Powers 2002: 799)

This definition illustrates that empirical knowledge derives from several studies of interventions *over time* rather than from the aggregate of practitioners' individual single systems or case-by-case evaluations of effectiveness. It is the aggregate of studies of trials of a treatment or intervention on whole groups or populations selected on the same criteria in which there are matched treatment and control groups where the researcher does not know who belongs to which group (termed double-blind RCTs). In evidence-based social work, the best available *knowledge* might include the accumulated knowledge built from evaluation and effectiveness studies, but this is not evidence-based practice. Such is the range of knowledge, which some believe is permissible in evidence-based social work, at least in principle, that it can include that generated through effectiveness and evaluation studies using qualitative *and* quantitative methods of enquiry, as well as practice knowledge. For evidence-based practice, however, quantitative enquiry, using RCTs and systematic reviews, is usually seen as the 'gold standard'. Even within social work, some argue that only studies employing RCTs should be included in SRs (Barber, in White 2008). The central evidence debate in social work revolves around the high-level legitimacy of quantitative, 'gold standard', experimental research and its tendency to sideline qualitative studies, as this excludes the bulk of interpretive social work research. As Soydan (2007: 3) notes, 'when it comes to measure the effects of social work interventions, experimental studies, especially when randomized, conducted very carefully, and large enough to generate statistical power, are the designs that are best fit for the purpose'.

Some proponents of evidence-based social work wish to move away from the idea that social workers use and build knowledge mainly from practice, where an eclectic range of theories and methods of intervention is used. As Mullen (2002) notes, eclecticism was a blind alley in the long road to evidence-based practice. Thus there is a difference between practice information, frontline experience, ideas about what works, practice knowledge, practice theory, and research-generated evidence as determined from replicable systematic reviews of accumulated research over time.

Social work has spent such a considerable part of its history trying to develop its own *theory* base – which has gone in myriad directions, from psychodynamic casework, to social groupwork, family therapy, community organization, cognitive behaviourism, and so on – that by the 1970s many wondered whether it was a unitary profession. It was at this point that the ecosystems perspective was offered as a unifying perspective, with problem-solving being essentially what client–worker relationships were about (Goldstein 1973). Advocates of eclecticism proposed a variety of intervention forms as a smorgasbord from which to choose, depending on the nature of the problem (Fischer 1978b). The idea was that the helping process be systematic, i.e., that it follow a rational process from assessment, to intervention, to evaluation, and that practitioners choose interventions with demonstrated effectiveness. In other words, practitioners had to use proven or empirically based interventions. Practice knowledge, or wisdom passed on by word of mouth or practice based on experience and practice wisdom, did not constitute knowledge, nor did knowledge not derived from systematic research form a reliable base on which to build practice.

Evidence-based social work, as we have noted, is presented as a process where evidence is used to inform decision-making where the onus is on the individual practitioner to locate the best available evidence (Gambrill 2006a; Gibbs and

Gambrill 2002). What sort of process it might be is discussed below, when we examine the differences and the relation between knowledge, evidence and information. Corcoran and Vandiver (in Roberts and Yeager 2006: 61) present a useful diagram of the way in which evidence, practice and professional consensus coalesce in providing resources for evidence-based practice (see Figure 1.1).

Evidence-based knowledge

Evidence-based knowledge, first referred to as 'knowledge-guided practice' and then more recently as 'best practice models', introduces the idea of an evidence hierarchy or continuum with 'gold standard' evidence at one extreme and experience, intuition and practice wisdom at the other (see Figure 1.2). Proponents of evidence-based knowledge equate evidence and knowledge. They hold that everything on the hierarchy or continuum counts as evidence, from 'gold standard'-derived knowledge to qualitative research (McNeece and Thyer 2004). Others include practice experience, intuition and practice wisdom (Roberts and Yeager 2004, 2006). They argue that different kinds and forms of knowledge are needed in social work practice and not just knowledge derived from scientific research. Hence 'best practices' are practice guidelines based on knowledge classified according to levels of empirical support, the evidence hierarchy – ranging from those based on research findings and, in the absence of available research, those based on professional consensus – and practitioner experience (see Rosen and Proctor 2003).

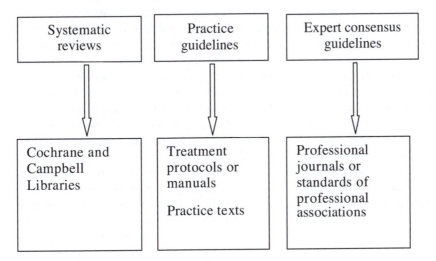

Figure 1.1 The relationship between evidence, practice and professional consensus.

Source: Corcoran and Vandiver (in Roberts and Yeager 2006: 61).

High reliability to directly inform practice

1.　Systematic reviews/meta-analyses

2.　Randomized controlled trials

3.　Quasi-experimental studies

4.　Case-control and cohort studies

5.　Pre-experimental group studies

6.　Surveys

7.　Qualitative studies

Low reliability

Figure 1.2 Evidence hierarchy.

Source: McNeece and Thyer (2004: 10).

As we observe in more detail in Chapter 6, best practice guidelines are system-atically developed statements to assist practitioners and clients in making decisions about appropriate interventions and or decisions in particular circumstances (Mullen *et al.* 2008). Howard and Jenson (1999: 283) claim that 'numerous studies indicate that guidelines can increase empirically based practice and improve clients' outcomes'. Gambrill (2006b) sees best practice guidelines as but one component of evidence-based practice, as is practitioner expertise. However, as with evidence-based practice, practice guidelines are not widely used in routine social work practice (Mullen *et al.* 2008; Mullen and Bacon 2004), so the same 'stuttering delay' referred to by Corcoran (2007) at the outset holds with evidence-based knowledge or best practice models.

In her review of Roberts and Yeager's (2004) *Evidence-based practice manual*, Lisa Rapp-Paglicci (2007: 427) claims that the authors use evidence-based knowledge to inform evidence-based practice. She describes it as a 'forerunner in evidence-based practice providing a multi-disciplinary approach inclusive of social work, psychology, public health, criminal justice, and medicine emphasizing the implementation of clinical best practices'. Like the term 'evidence-based practices' eschewed by Thyer (2008a), what exactly are 'clinical best practices'? The answer lies, perhaps, in the performative aspect of the verb 'best', in that it is assumed to be a standard of quality or excellence that is formally achieved as a consistent, measurable and durable performance of practice. But no researcher has ever measured 'best practices'. What is most revealing is that it is unlikely that a social worker would define herself as a 'best practice' practitioner because it is a benchmark of quality within policy discourse that leaves the actual practice of the social worker remote and at a distance. Therefore, 'best practice' guidelines or protocols do not actually ever represent the real-life, concrete practices of the social worker.

Contested knowledge: what the philosophers have to say

In laying out the material thus far around various normative definitions and key terms associated with evidence-based practice, this chapter has largely treated 'knowledge' and the interface between 'knowledge' and 'evidence' – at least as portrayed in the literature on evidence-based social work, where they are generally seen as unproblematic constructs – with some reservation. The remaining sections of this chapter begin to develop the critical stance that is signalled in the subtitle of this book as a creative exploration of various parameters and positions within the evidence-based practice program and in developing arguments *against* certain variants of evidence-based practice as they attempt to mobilize their way into social work.

In plain terms, evidence is a form of knowledge. But, as we shall see, it is *just* that. Evidence is only one form of knowledge among many. So, more broadly, what is knowledge? We may begin with a few preliminary observations. First, socially, technically and conceptually, we are framed by knowledge. As Messer-Davidow *et al.* (1993: vii) observe, knowledge helps us to produce our world and our understanding of it. Knowledge specifies the objects we may study and the relations that obtain among them. It provides our criteria for explanations – of truth, significance and impact – and conceptual frameworks and methods, such as quantification, interpretation and analysis that regulate our access to an understanding of the social world. Second, knowledge produces practitioners, orthodox and heterodox, specialist and generalist, theoretical and experimental. Third, it produces 'economies of value' (*ibid.*). It manufactures plentiful discourse around refereed journal articles, conference papers, detailed monographs, prize-winning books, and much debate and discussion. Knowledge also generates prestige, institutional research rankings, and scientific and scholarly research stars.

Steve Fuller (1993) has shown how philosophers have a great deal to say about different forms of knowledge. The branch of philosophy that deals critically with the status and forms of knowledge is called 'epistemology'. Indeed, much of the debate and dialogue in the social sciences broadly, and in social work in particular, are steeped in a rich heritage of philosophical discourse about the nature of knowledge. Drawing on a longstanding but contested terrain of knowledge called the 'philosophy of science', Fuller is concerned with the way in which the boundaries between science and non-science have emerged over the past century. It is our contention that this sort of boundary work is being played out in the secondary field of evidence-based practice as it gets formulated in social work. Philosophers of science, Fuller (1993: 134–135) argues, have sought '*demarcation criteria* that systematically discriminate the sciences from non-scientific (and especially pseudo-scientific, such as alternative health therapies) forms of knowledge' and 'have drawn the science–nonscience boundary largely to cast aspersions on the legitimacy of particular pretenders to the title of science'. However, Fuller concludes that this boundary work is a rhetorical one, since philosophers of science have failed to discover any properties common to the sciences in general and hence any 'ahistorical' essence that can be bounded (see also Smith 1987).

One particular camp in the contested field of knowledge in the philosophy of sciences that has played a particularly virulent role in the boundary-making, and one that has a direct impact on the formation of the evidence-based practice program, is positivism. For those readers who are unfamiliar with positivism, it claims that knowledge can only come from affirmation of theories through the strict scientific method. In philosophy of science terms, it argues that all true knowledge is ultimately scientific and that all things are ultimately measurable. Positivism combines with empiricism in claiming that observational evidence is indispensable for knowledge of the world. It is our contention that the re-emergent scientism that is taking place in social work around the evidence-based practice debate is essentially derived from a positivistic stance. Indeed, Bruce Thyer (2008b: 339), one of the main advocates of a positivistic approach to social work, published an article subtitled 'We are all positivists!' claiming that the 'evidence-based practice movement provides the field with a wonderful opportunity to dramatically increase the extent to which professional activities in the realms of policy and practice can be more solidly grounded in scientific research'. Positivism contends that social sciences should mimic the natural sciences as part of the boundary delimitation discussed above.

Positivists distinguish theory from observation. It is for this reason that many advocates of evidence-based social work argue strongly for a reduction in theorizing and an increase in empirical research, which rests on establishing 'observational truths', e.g., about 'what works'. However, the distinction between observation and theory is meaningless. Philosopher Hilary Putnam argues that the dichotomy of observational terms and theoretical terms is the problem from which to start. Putnam (1999: 25) demonstrates this with four objections:

1 Something is referred to as 'observational' if it is observable directly with our senses. Then an observational term cannot be applied to something unobservable. If this is the case, there are no observational terms.
2 Some unobservable terms are not even theoretical and belong to neither observational terms nor theoretical terms. Some theoretical terms refer primarily to observational terms.
3 Reports of observational terms frequently contain theoretical terms.
4 A scientific theory may not contain any theoretical terms and an example of this is Darwin's original theory of evolution.[2]

Within the philosophy of science and the social sciences over the past fifty years, it has generally been accepted that positivism embodies a fundamental misunderstanding of social reality, that it is ahistorical, depoliticized and an inappropriate application of theoretical concepts. It is argued that positivism systematically fails to appreciate the extent to which the so-called world of observational facts it yielded does not exist 'out there' in the objective world, but is itself a product of socially and historically mediated human consciousness. Moreover, positivism has consistently ignored the role of the 'observer' in the constitution of social reality and failed to take account of the historical and social conditions affecting the representation of observations.[3] One of the leading critical theorists, Habermas (1968), makes a stronger accusation that positivism has had a pernicious effect on society at large. In his work on the 'colonization of the life-world', he claims that scientistic modes of decision-making and method have encroached so much into the public sphere that a dominant 'technical rationality' has become all pervasive, overtaking all other forms of social rationality. Habermas also highlights the way that positivism ignored major findings of Enlightenment philosophers:

> Positivism turned its back to the theory of knowledge, whose philosophical self-liquidation had been carried on by Hegel and Marx, who were of one mind in this regard. In so doing, positivism regressed behind the level of reflection once attained by Kant.
>
> (Habermas 1968: 121)

In *Truth and method* (1989), Hans Georg Gadamer, a distinguished German philosopher, accuses positivism of being not only illusory but also an unnecessary distraction within the human sciences. Further on in this book, we ask the same question as to whether evidence-based practice is an unnecessary distraction in social work. Gadamer draws a distinction between *techne* and *praxis*. While the former is representative of the scientific mode of thinking concerning itself with technical skills and an individual's skilful mastery of them, and can be learned, *praxis* involves knowledge about human beings, especially human action, and carries a moral dimension to it, since individual action connects a researcher with other human beings. Gadamer (1989: 317) says that 'we learn a *techne* and can also forget it. But we do not learn moral knowledge, nor can we forget it.' This is why *praxis*, unlike its opposite *techne*, always involves a 'concern' for other beings, and thus underscores the need for moral judgement. On Gadamer's reading, since the positivistic sciences, like some variants of evidence-based practice, are essentially derived from *techne*, at the expense of *praxis*, they show no ethical concern for other human beings and are, therefore, immoral.

Against the attempts of positivists to influence social sciences, well-known British sociologist Anthony Giddens (1976: 13) remarked that 'Those who still wait for a Newton of social sciences are not only waiting for a train that won't arrive, they're in the wrong station altogether'. For Giddens, social work and the social sciences are based on an interpretivist philosophy of science that marks a fundamental difference between the sciences and non-sciences such that human behaviour, unlike atoms and molecules, can only be understood from the insider's perspective, in terms of the interpretation of meanings that actors employ. As Martyn Jones (1990: 188) argued, social work is bound up with the fact that practitioners and clients are pervasive interpreters of others as well as themselves. Thus the positivist claims for social work treat clients as little more than a factor that complicates interventions by making them less well behaved than billiard balls. Howe (2004: 54) is even more scathing when he observes that evidence-based practice:

> ... elevates quantitative-experimental methods to the top of the methodological hierarchy and constrains qualitative methods to a largely auxiliary role in pursuit of the *technocratic* aim of accumulating knowledge of 'what works' ... 'what works' is not an innocent notion. Concrete instances of the claim 'Intervention *I* works' are elliptical for instances of the claim 'Intervention *I* works to accomplish outcome *O*'. The desired outcomes are embraced as more valuable than other possible outcomes.

In line with Gadamer's defintion of *techne*, and Habermas's critique of 'technical rationality', Howe concludes that 'the aim of determining "what works" is *technocratic*; it focuses on the question of whether evidence-based interventions are effective in achieving *given* outcomes' (*ibid.*).

Information- or evidence-based?

As noted above, the positivist approach to evidence refers to proven and rigorously validated facts based on observation, which support a conclusion, statement or outcome. It refers to 'its common usage *in science* to distinguish data from theory' (Sherman 2003: 7 emphasis added). But a great deal of confusion is generated by the overlapping use of the terms 'evidence', 'theory', 'information' and 'knowledge'. Scott-Findlay and Pollock (2004) note that often the terms 'research' and 'knowledge' are used as synonyms for 'evidence', when in science the term 'evidence' has long been understood to mean the findings of empirical research, i.e., systematic data and RCT studies.

For purists, recent attempts to broaden the definition of evidence to include clinical experience and experiential or experience-based knowledge have been misleading, serving only to add to the confusion about what constitutes evidence. *Broadening understanding of the basis for clinical decision-making and conceptualizing evidence are quite different tasks.* Other factors, not other forms of evidence, shape the decision-making process, but they are not evidence. We might better term them 'information processes'. Confusing evidence with other factors has hindered research and the improvement of clinical decision-making in healthcare. Scott-Findlay and Pollock (2004) argue that this confusion results from the ambiguous use of the term 'evidence'. They argue for specificity in the use of the term 'evidence' and urge the restriction of this term to research findings. This perspective runs contrary to the all-inclusive approach advocated by Gambrill and others in social work. While acknowledging the importance of other influences, including knowledge, on the decision-making process, Scott-Findlay and Pollock (2004) insist that they are not evidence. Personal experience, experiential knowledge and service user involvement must be valued for what they are. They should not have to be disguised as 'types of evidence' to be deemed to have value. Being specific to language, the goal is to improve decision-making by increasing practitioners' reliance on research findings, i.e., evidence, while acknowledging and valuing the important part played by other forms of knowledge or information in the decision-making process.

The distinctions are important, especially if one considers Charlton's (1997) observation that evidence, i.e., research data, is of no value to practitioners unless it is translated into usable information. This, however, leads to the possibility that we are really witnessing an information-based rather than an evidence-based practice. It strikes us that much of what gets talked about as evidence-based practice may, in fact, turn out to be little more than information-based practice, such that guidelines and protocols for evidence at the point of reception on the desk of a frontline social worker are actually conceived as 'information reports'. These reports involve the information processing of data and, in the broadest sense, the storage, retrieval and processing of data becomes an essential resource for social work decision-making. As Machlup (1983: 642) has noted, the original meaning of the word 'information' derives from the Latin *informare*, which means 'to put into form'. Crucially, information involves data that are processed and considered to be useful. Evidence-based guidelines often look very much like styles of information reports that are *factive* in form. Moreover, we are not dealing with something that resembles an interface between knowledge and evidence, as some advocates of evidence-based practice suggest, but rather with the interface between evidence and information. If we examine the distinction between knowledge and information given by Machlup (1983), it is easy to discern that it is information that is the key coupling term to evidence and not knowledge. We have seen above how knowledge is highly contestable. Generally, 'information' and 'knowledge' are distinguished along three axes:

1 *Multiplicity*: Information is piecemeal, fragmented and particular. Knowledge is structured, coherent and universal.
2 *Temporality*: Information is timely, transitory and even ephemeral. Knowledge is enduring and temporally expansive.
3 *Spatiality*: Information is a flow across spaces. Knowledge is a stock, specifically located, yet spatially expansive.

In summary, information is conceived of as a process, whereas knowledge is a state (Machlup 1983: 642). Having an understanding is different from having information. Understanding is an interpolative and judgemental process. It is cognitive and analytical. It is the process by which we take information and synthesize new information from previously held understanding. The difference between understanding and information is the difference between 'learning' and 'memorizing'. Thus it is a concern to us that if the emphasis is on information-gathering and processing, we are witnessing a shift in social work away from learning towards procedural organizational memory. Crucially with evidence-based practice, we are dealing with information, or more accurately, informational processes that rest on considerations of utility. The utility of the information is based on spatial and temporal flows, the content of which is often fragmented and provisional. In this sense, we wonder whether, should the advocates of evidence-based practice be successful, it is more likely that social work will come to resemble information-based rather than evidence-based practice?

But we live in an 'information age', where we are bombarded with information, and practitioners need considerable experience, professional expertise and strong critical appraisal skills to discern good information from bad. When faced with a health problem, the choices might range from herbal remedies to fancy gadgets, to massage and aromatherapy, conventional medical treatment and drug therapy, to a range of strangely named psychotherapies, and so on, such that it is extremely difficult to discern what works – evidence – other than by trial and error – practice knowledge.

Advocates of evidence-based practice are adamant that it is not enough, nor is it ethically appropriate, to base decisions about interventions and/or treatments on flimsy *information*, such as individuals' experience of what works for them. Word-of-mouth or misleading media reports or inconclusive research reported in the media do not constitute evidence. The best evidence derives from systematic reviews using meta-synthesis of RCTs with objective findings of the effectiveness of interventions across contexts and over time.

'Best available evidence', then, reflects a realist or pragmatic approach to evidence, acknowledging that, more often than not, in social work anyway, pure evidence from SRs of RCT studies is not available. All that we have to go on is the best available evidence at the time, which may or may not include RCTs. In the absence of 'gold-standard' evidence, quasi-experimental, social intervention research, qualitative case and participatory action research studies, and so on, constitute *the best available evidence at the time*.

It is important to understand that evidence-based practice is not merely about decision-making or the application of particular research studies to practice. It is not empirical practice, or choosing from lists of empirically supported treatments (ESTs) or interventions (ESIs), or research-based practice. It is not about encouraging practitioners to make use of psychosocial interventions supported by credible outcomes or to evaluate clinical outcomes using single-system designs (Reid 1994). Nor is it about practice information, based on experience, practice wisdom or intuition (Soydan 2007). Information based on individual or aggregated experience does not constitute knowledge nor does knowledge constitute evidence, as strictly defined. There is much confusion within social work, however, because advocates of evidence-based knowledge tend to equate evidence and knowledge (Roberts and Yeager 2004, 2006).

A narrow definition of knowledge is adopted in the evidence-based practice discourse that often amounts to a simplistic reduction to information, i.e., empirically untested knowledge or factual data. Hence, often evidence-based practice is not really about knowledge production and transfer but rather about information storage, retrieval and reporting and the way in which information systems are managed and processed (Castells 2002). As noted by Gambrill (in Thyer and Kazi 2004: 217), '[e]vidence-based practice requires the free flow of information'. But '[p]reparing rigorous appraisals of practice-related research findings and making them accessible to all involved parties is a key aim of evidence-based practice' (*ibid.*: 218). Hence care must be taken not to reduce evidence-based practice to the simple diagram of 'information = decision' rather than 'evidence via systematic reviews = knowledge on which to base decisions' within a culture and networks which formalize processes so derived.

A process of formalization

As already noted, this book claims that evidence-based practice is not simply about the application of research in practice or how social workers use evidence to make evaluative judgements or complex decisions. It is crucially about the broader, macro institutional and policy environment, which is driving evidence-based policy and practice, and its ramifications for those involved in knowledge production and research. At its extreme, it advocates that only knowledge derived over time from RCTs constitutes evidence on which to base policy and practice. At the mezzo level, this then drives the formal professional networks, organizational systems and practice cultures in which researchers and practitioners are embedded, and the best practice guidelines and the models of implementation which authorize and regulate what social workers are permitted to do. It is a form of technical rationalism that sets the normative requirements of practice in order to stamp out any vestiges of ideological or critical enquiry or professional autonomy or authority-based practice (Gambrill 1999, 2001, 2006b) which have long been the province of the social sciences and anti-oppressive social work practice. It might be useful here to think of levels of formalization:

1 At the *macro level*, evidence-based policy drives organizational cultures within research and practice.
2 At the *mezzo level*, this drives professional, agency- or community-based practice.
3 At the *micro level*, the individual practitioner makes decisions.

We need to understand that, at the micro level, individual practitioners do not make decisions in a vacuum but in a complex web of relationships within a broad, macro political landscape. They are actors in networks and conduits through which information flows, as determined *inter alia* by macro policies – including the policies of the organizations they work for, government policy relating to the clients they deal with and the way these factors prescribe the nature of the work that they do – which are increasingly inimical to their professional values and training. Increasingly that work is procedural and takes place in a managerial risk-saturated practice environment (Webb 2006). More widely, evidence-based practice, outcomes-based interventions and 'what works' are embedded in a climate of political opinion which surrounds the formation of social policy in advanced capitalist societies and the systems of quality assurance and performance culture associated with the process. As Elliott (2001) shows, they can be summarized as follows:

1   Social practices are activities which need to be justified as an *effective* and *efficient* means of producing desirable outputs.
2   Means and ends are contingently related. What constitutes an appropriate means for bringing about the ends-in-view needs to be determined on the basis of *empirical evidence*.
3   The determination of means requires a clear and precise pre-specification of ends as tangible and measurable outputs or targets, which constitute the *quality standards* against which the performance of social practitioners is to be judged.

It is readily apparent that the prevailing context in social work tends to reflect these assumptions, inasmuch as it prioritizes *target-setting* alongside forms of evaluation and quality assurance. These are benchmarked against performance measures of interventions and against *indicators* of success in achieving targets. We can see how evidence-based practice lends itself neatly to treating social work interventions as manipulative devices for securing desired levels of 'what works' outputs.

   Individual social workers do not usually locate and decide on permissible and admissible evidence on which to base practice. An intermediary process occurs in which their agencies determine myriad prescriptive policies, including codes of conduct, which are increasingly over-riding professional codes of ethics, and best practice guidelines variously and mostly loosely based on existing knowledge or evidence-based practice (see Gambrill 2006a). The practitioner's decision is linked to a complex set of steering factors derived from a 'networked evidence system' promoted within neo-liberal and managerial institutional and organizational cultures. Thus, for example, mental health practice takes place within an institutional culture which changes over time: the most recent major change has been de-institutionalization brought on by economic rationalist drivers that it was less costly to care for people in the community. A second major cultural driver in mental health is the diagnostic classification system that is vigorously promoted as a way of standardizing assessment and intervention regimes. Most recently, a major factor influencing practice is evidence-based policy based on effectiveness studies employing rigorous experimental research. To justify our claim that evidence-based practice in social work is best characterized as an 'emerging actor network', it is necessary to analyze the complex pathways of formalization that have embedded it within our professional, institutional and organizational cultures, as we do in Chapters 4 and 5.

   One of the major factors that led to the evidence-based practice movement is those developments in information technology from which actor network theory derives. Competing now with professional means of knowledge production and dissemination is the information highway. Paradoxically, however, evidence-based practice has arisen as a kind of 'quality check' on the enormous amount of information that is available to policy-makers and potential service users. It has led to a distrusting stance towards professionals once credited with expertise and authority by virtue of their professional education and vast knowledge, skill and experience. In a sense, by slapping a quality check on this information, professionals reclaim their turf because it is they who generate the research and the practice that constitute evidence-based practice. Not just any old information accessible via the internet will suffice but only that which results from solid, scientific research. Thus the profession of social work uses evidence-based practice to defend its turf, to generate its own evidence and to stay abreast of the big boys and girls in evidence-based medicine and nursing, and so on. It has to play the game to stay in the game. It has had to, through peer pressure, adopt a 'what works' agenda. So social work operates within a broader network of other professions and occupations, adopting, as it goes, some of their cultures and practices. Despite its vigorous attempts to develop its own knowledge base, social work has always been a derivative discipline inextricably linked to the broader social and behavioural science and health disciplines, as well as law, political science, and so on.

Social work is, then, a conduit of information that often comes from above – including agency hierarchies, practice protocols, organizational policies – and below the clients and communities that social workers deal with, and from within their professional and organizational cultures and without – the external influences impinging on social work. Often social workers are caught in the middle trying to hold onto what little autonomy they have, to make evaluative judgements and decisions in the moment. As we shall see in Chapter 6, research on decision-making heuristics shows that, despite all the information and evidence, social workers still make decisions based on their in-the-moment intuitive judgements or what Varela (1999) calls 'readiness for action'. So intricately connected are we to a chain of action and reaction that we only become aware of the sequence of events that led to a decision once we move into reflective, after-the-action mode (Gray 2007).

What, then, are the implications of social workers being 'actors in a network' or chain of decisions and events? Social network analysis is a powerful tool for analyzing these connections in everyday practice and their impact on social workers' decisions and actions. It asks that they reflect on who it is that they speak and listen to, on who or what it is that influences their thinking. It could be a book that they have just read, a movie that they have just seen, a conversation that they have just had with a colleague or friend, an internet site that they have just visited, or a systematic review that they have just read. The possibilities are endless. More broadly, however, we are concerned with how evidence-based practice assumes prominence. Who are the actors or change agents and what are their networks? Which professor visited which university and when? How did the idea of single-system design get from the USA to the UK? Why does the 'empirical clinical practice model' not get translated to the UK? Why is clinical social work a major player in the USA and not in the UK? These are big questions and one is tempted to answer them in a general fashion, noting the preponderance of social work academics in the USA who have a strong grounding in psychology, especially behaviourism and cognitivism, while UK academics seem to be grounded in sociology and social policy. Even the schools in which they work and the programs in which they teach are different, depending on which side of the world they are on. While we might want to trace the beginnings of evidence-based practice to social work's beginnings and include the effectiveness movement *en route*, we need to realize that the 'evidence turn' marks a distinct break with empirical clinical and practitioner–researcher practice models in the USA and with the practice evaluation movement in the UK. As Mullen (2002) noted, these were diversions and dead-ends but the path to which they pointed was a road that inevitably would be taken, though reluctantly by some and avoided by others.

Social work's reception of evidence-based practice

The reception of evidence-based practice in social work is a key consideration throughout the rest of this book. We shall see that the uptake of evidence-based practice has not been uniform and the application of research to practice has been, at best, erratic and unsystematic, and, some might say, almost non-existent. For example, according to Gambrill (in Thyer and Kazi 2004: 217), '[p]resent-day practices in social work do not have characteristics of evidence-based practice as envisioned by its originators'. It seems that the closer one is to the inner circle of the medical professions where evidence-based medicine arose, the more intense the uptake. Of the 'outer edge disciplines' (Trinder, in Trinder and Reynolds 2000: 14) which have lagged behind, social work has been slowest. Not only has social work lagged behind other professional disciplines in generating evidence, via RCTs of its interventions, but it has also under-utilized scientific knowledge. The slow uptake of evidence-based practice, not only in social work but also throughout the health and human services, continues to lead to a 'discrepancy between what research has demonstrated to be effective and what is actually … occurring in practice' (Mullen *et al*. 2008: 1; see also Mullen and Bacon 2004; Weissman and Sanderson 2001). There is clearly not a continuous link between knowledge production and its implementation, as we show in Chapter 6. Thus the use of evidence-based practice in contemporary social work intervention is limited (Gambrill 2006b; Mullen and Bacon 2004). Why is this?

Many have argued that the regimes of evidence-based practice exclude valuable forms of qualitative inquiry which get much closer to understanding the lived experience of people beset with problems. Equally important is the meaning they attach to these experiences. The counter argument, however, is that the researcher's main purpose is not to understand problems but to solve them using the 'best evidence' available at the time, based on sound research rather than freely available information, as outlined above. Social workers' reluctance to engage in experimental research has seen them lag behind medical science and behavioural psychology, where double-blind clinical trials have become routine. Instead, social workers argue that their circumstances are too complex and problematic for reductive experimental methods, hence social work's 'research exceptionalism'. Some go so far as to say that many US social workers are not much interested in empirical evidence of any kind (David Stoesz, personal communication 23 May 2008). Stoesz, therefore, worries that 'best evidence' equates to qualitative studies, dressed up in postmodern regalia, decorated with alternative epistemologies and coloured with subjugated voices, which are structured and carried out in such a way that affirms professional ideology. The result is a romantic, non-replicable, self-affirming discourse with little empirical foundation. Critical reviews of qualitative research in social work point to weak methodology, small sample sizes, low reliability, and so on (Shek *et al.* 2005).

However, social research generally has to balance concerns about knowledge production with knowledge utility or relevance. The latter has been the province of applied research and the former the preoccupation of basic or 'pure' research, loosely non-university and university-based research respectively (Hammersley 2003). The former is generally accorded lower status than the latter. But as we have seen in relation to evidence-based policy, in recent years 'there has been an increasing push toward valuing the applied end of the spectrum' (Hammersley 2003: 29). This is articulated by knowledge-production theorists as 'Mode 2' research, which is distinguishable from the 'Mode 1' academic model (Gibbons 2000; Gibbons *et al.* 1994). Mode 2 research:

1 focuses on solving problems arising in particular practical contexts, where the aim is to generate a solution or a product, rather than simply to contribute to a body of knowledge;
2 takes place via teamwork, with teams being 'non-hierarchical' and 'essentially transient';
3 is 'transdisciplinary' in orientation; research teams are interdisciplinary, and, while disciplinary knowledge is drawn on, what is most important is the knowledge, understanding and techniques accumulated through experience in doing Mode 2 research;
4 is practical in character, with accountability involving users as well as researchers. Market considerations can be crucial: its products are likely to be judged, at least in part, by whether they are 'competitive' and 'cost effective' (Hammersley 2003).

There have been many attempts in social work to combine these seemingly disparate approaches, which is where Hammersley (2003) sees action research, with its dual concern for discovering the facts and social improvement, in its various forms, entering the equation. But evidence-based practice sharply distinguishes research from other forms of activity. As Hammersley (2003: 34) notes, research is a specialized form of inquiry where the goal is the production of knowledge. Hence it is at odds with action and intervention research, 'conceptualized as the whole process of devising solutions to practical problems, implementing them, monitoring outcomes, formulating better solutions, and so on, in a spiral of improvement'. While there is an element of inquiry involved, it is *inquiry-subordinated-to-a-practical-activity* and hence not research. Since research is objective inquiry, it cannot be partisan and have liberatory goals. This is not to say that research might not contribute to political goals or social improvement, merely that such ends are not its primary purpose. Hence one might draw a distinction between evidence-based practice weighted towards pure quantitative-experimental methodology and evidence-based social work favouring applied qualitative-interpretive methods (see Table 1.1). These distinctions will become clearer in the chapters which follow, as we seek to correct some of the myths surrounding evidence-based practice.

Table 1.1 Distinction between evidence-based practice and evidence-based social work methodologies

Pure quantitative-experimental	*Applied qualitative-interpretivist*
Scientific or academic – tries to maintain distance from the phenomenon under study and attaches high importance to validity and reliability	Practical – assumes a close relationship between research and practice or policy-making and attaches high importance to relevance
Basic – generates and explores hypotheses	Applied and addresses and meets a felt need
Experimental 'gold standard' research methodology – RCTs and SRs	Naturalistic forms of enquiry, such as in-depth interviews, focus groups and conversations or narratives
Measurement or numerically based	Text based – unit of analysis is transcripts from interviews, focus groups, conversations, personal narratives, client stories, etc.
Decontextualized	Contextualized or context-based
Not directly designed to feed into processes of decision-making	Directly designed to feed into processes of decision-making
Audience is fellow researchers, constituting a community of organized skepticism, who make judgements as to the validity of the research by employing the burden of proof	Audience is consumers, whether practitioners, service users or policy-makers, who will judge the validity of the research on its utility and instrumentality
Concerned with contributing to a cumulative body of knowledge	Concerned with utility and relevance, with the provision of knowledge of immediate practical use
Emphasizes the researcher's autonomous role in choice of research topic and methodology	Dedicated or democratic, practical research where participation of those being researched is deemed important to the relevance of the findings

Adapted from Hammersley (2003).

Correcting some myths

In this penultimate section, we begin to correct some of the myths surrounding evidence-based practice as a way of laying the foundation for our more detailed treatment of each of these in the chapters that follow. It will be instructive to the reader to consider the myths surrounding evidence-based practice as they engage with some of the more nuanced and detailed analysis that follows in later chapters.

Myth 1: empiricism is the only way of knowing

Empiricism is simply one way of knowing that is appropriate for certain questions – such as: does it work? – but not for others (Corcoran 2007: 548). There is much in social work that is not within the purview of science *per se*, such as values and ethics, diversity, the history of social welfare, policy and so on. However, we should desist from teaching students practice techniques – and the knowledge informing them – where empirical research has shown that they do not work or are actively harmful to clients.

Myth 2: evidence-based practice is an epistemology

Evidence-based practice is not an epistemology or theory of knowledge or a way of knowing. It is a system for practice that is based on a program of formalization, albeit based on certain epistemological assumptions, where the central focus is knowledge gained via *empirical research* using the *empirical method*. Its pivotal argument is that evidence is *empirical* or *empirically based*, i.e., the outcome of systematic, scientific research which, in its narrowest sense, employs a positivistic methodology with RCTs as the 'gold standard'. It is accumulated over time, as successive studies replicate the findings of prior research thus establishing the legitimacy of particular interventions.

Myth 3: if we provide the evidence, practitioners will apply it

Just because the evidence is there, does not mean that it will be used. As Corcoran (2007: 50) notes, it is likely to take longer than we think to get practitioners to use evidence-based practice. Practitioners have been quick to point out the limitations of evidence-based practice in dealing with complex, situated practice issues, as has the 'qualitative research community', whom Staller (2006: 503) implores to resist evidence-based practice in favour of a focus on practice-based evidence (PBE). She claims that PBE:

> ... changes the nature of [the] debate, highlights the practitioner role, recog-nizes practitioner agency in evaluating evidence, focuses on real-world situations (thus embracing complications), and honors the notion of multiple and competing evidence sources. PBE encourages research designs favored by

qualitative researchers that explore contextually situated practices and promote value-based social justice agendas.

Myth 4: the proper pursuit of knowledge is always conducive to improved practice

As Hammersley (2003) notes, first we cannot assume that our practical and political commitments, however laudable, will necessarily have a desirable impact on the pursuit of inquiry any more than we can assume that because a researcher has objectionable beliefs or unacceptable political allegiances, the findings produced will be false. Bias is an ever-present danger in all research. It is not restricted to those who have commitments we disagree with. No one who does research lacks attitudes towards the issues being investigated, and usually they will not be without concerns about the consequences of their work. Further, however politically progressive these commitments are, they may still distort the process of inquiry. Second, we cannot assume that producing knowledge about an issue is always likely to lead to an improvement in the situation, or that inquiry is always an essential requirement for significant improvement, or that producing knowledge about an issue is always the best way to achieve change. While not denying the practical value of research, it is not automatic. Producing sound knowledge about an issue does not *always* lead to improvement or desirable change. Indeed, sometimes it can make the situation worse, at least temporarily (see also Hammersley 2002).

Myth 5: evidence-based practice is only a medical model

While evidence-based practice originated in medicine, it is incorrect to say that the approach which derived from it is a 'medical model' of practice. Evidence-based practice does not say anything about the aetiology of problems (e.g., biological), the default mode of treatment (e.g., drugs or surgery) or the default providers of care (e.g., physicians). These positions constitute the medical model. By way of contrast, evidence-based practice outlines a scientific model useful in health and social care disciplines that claim to base their practices on scientific research. The fact that evidence-based practice emerged from medicine does not make it a medical model, even though evidence-based practice has been embraced by many *health practice disciplines*, like nursing, medicine, occupational therapy, psychology, dentistry and psychiatry, whose research training is often minimal.

Myth 6: evidence-based practice exclusively involves applying evidence to decision-making

Sackett *et al.*'s (1996) original, over-quoted definition of evidence-based practice has stuck like Superglue when most contemporary writers and thinkers have advanced beyond the evidence–decision interface to a much more comprehensive approach to practice which involves evidence, practitioner judgement and client values. This tripartite alliance makes for far greater complexity in the way in which problems are framed, evidence is collected and shared with clients, and clients participate in decisions that follow.

Conclusion

In this opening chapter, we have clarified the key terms used in the discourse on evidence-based practice, begun to develop a critical stance against certain variants of this discourse and attempted to correct some misconceptions about it. We have seen how, within evidence-based social work, the findings of systematically generated research should be applied. It represents the farthest-reaching and most direct and concerted attempt to prescribe and predetermine the actions of social workers, as well as to shape professional identity around a resurgent scientism. Chapter 2 critically examines the methodology of evidence-based practice. The approach taken lends itself more closely to a process by which evidence-based practice becomes standardized, that does not necessarily follow a sequential unfolding of events or entities, nor is it necessarily about 'what works' but rather 'what counts as research' (Lincoln and Cannella 2004: 6). Hence Chapter 2 examines what lies behind evidence-based practice and represents an attempt to understand the broader processes that embed it, such as *inter alia* a return to 'methodological conservatism' (Lincoln and Cannella 2004), 'reemergent scientism' (Maxwell 2004) or 'neoclassical experimentalism' (Howe 2004). Like Timmermans and Berg (2003: 8), we argue that evidence-based practice 'is part of a wider movement to generate uniformity and quality control by streamlining processes'.

Notes

1 Sometimes referred to as 'randomized field trials' or 'randomized clinical trials'.
2 http://en.wikipedia.org/wiki/Logical_positivism
3 http://en.wikipedia.org/wiki/Positivism

2 The 'gold standard' of evidence

This chapter sets out what has come to be regarded as the 'gold standard' approach to evidence-based practice, as it is derived from medical science, pioneered by David Sackett (Sackett *et al.* 1996, 1997, 2000). It is concerned with demonstrating to the reader how evidence-based practice is operationalized at different levels in gathering, reviewing and disseminating research findings, with the purpose of informing policy and practice. We use case examples from current Cochrane and Campbell Collaboration reviews to familiarize the reader with what has come to be known as the 'gold standard' methodology. This approach is entrenched in a modernist model of science that may be appropriate for the physical sciences, but which has struggled to establish wide applicability in the social sciences, particularly when interpretivist ways of understanding human social life have been a competing influence. Bruce Thyer (2006: 36) outlines five steps involved in an evidence-based practice approach to social work:

1 Convert one's need for information into an answerable question.
2 Track down the best clinical evidence to answer that question.
3 Critically appraise the evidence in terms of its validity, clinical significance and usefulness.
4 Integrate this critical appraisal of research evidence with one's clinical expertise and patient values and circumstances.
5 Evaluate one's effectiveness and efficiency in undertaking the four previous steps and strive for self-improvement.

These steps offer a reasonable and appropriate guide for frontline practice, but leave room for a range of methods in moving through the steps. The 'gold standard' approach to fulfilling these steps has adopted a particular definition of 'best evidence' in Step 2 in terms of an experimental research design. The process of critical appraisal in Step 3 has been standardized in a particular approach to systematic reviews and meta-analysis of research literature. The evidence-based practice process has been aligned with standardized procedures and the favouring of particular research methodologies, which are examined in this chapter. The scrutiny of research findings for their rigour and validity and the systematic compilation of these findings culminate in the production of 'best practice guidelines' based on 'proven' diagnostic and effective intervention knowledge, which may then be distributed to clinicians (Gould and Kendall 2007; Mullen *et al.* 2008; Roberts and Yeager 2006). Such guidelines offer procedural instructions on which interventions are in order, when to provide interventions, how long the intervention should be, and other details about effectiveness in making decisions about the care of service users. We discuss how, typically, a group of research experts evaluate the scientific literature according to a set of criteria based on a 'hierarchy of evidence' and then offer recommendations based on the strength of the evidence aimed at frontline practitioners. According to the 'gold standard' of evidence-based practice, best practice guidelines should be derived from scientific evidence, preferably a meta-analysis of randomized clinical trials and other experimental designs which offer probability estimates of each outcome (Soydan 2008). The Cochrane Collaboration leads and promotes the philosophy of 'gold standard' evidence for healthcare decision-making, claiming that 'Cochrane reviews represent the highest level of evidence on which to base clinical treatment decisions' (Cochrane Collaboration nd: 1).

This selective and standardized approach to evidence-based practice is not, however, without controversy. The quality of evidence and the nature of effectiveness are central issues in this controversy. The dominant approach to the systematic review of evidence favours the meta-analysis of the results of randomized controlled trials (RCTs) conceptualized as the 'gold standard' in evidence of effectiveness, with other experimental designs ranked as lower in quality. Hence the results of qualitative, interpretive and critical research are generally not regarded as evidence. If qualitative research is recognized, findings may be used to enhance understanding of results from experimental studies, rather than as being useful in their own right. The prevailing privilege of experimental designs, the RCT and quantitative research in evidence-based practice is in conflict with the newer interpretive and participatory paradigms for research. These paradigms have influenced a range of research approaches popular in social work efforts to generate knowledge for practice. Advocates of the 'gold standard', however, argue that only the RCT offers strong evidence and definitive answers about cause and effect, which is needed as evidence of effectiveness.

This chapter offers a critique of the behaviourist–decisionist epistemology[1] that has developed around evidence-based practice. That is, the way in which a methodological approach has endorsed the decisions for practitioners in a way that gives validity to the method devised by expert authority rather than the content or context of the practice decision. We consider whether the evidence-based practice 'gold standard' approach is about 'what works' for real clients in real practice contexts or whether it is about establishing among the realm of experts 'what counts as evidence'.

Proponents of experimental evidence are wary of reasoning from basic principles or experience. They distrust claims based on professional authority and expertise or opinion-based models of intervention (Gambrill 1999, 2006a). They prefer to remain agnostic as to the reason why something should or should not work and aim to measure objectively whether or not an intervention works in controlled settings.

Systematic methodologies to develop best practice guidelines have emerged. Hierarchies and techniques to rate the scientific quality of research findings are applied and statistical meta-analyses are used to aggregate the results of multiple trial interventions. It is intended that the results of these meta-analyses will be the basis for the development of best practice guidelines. In addition, cost–benefit data are increasingly included in the evidence upon which the guidelines are based. Relying on formal analytic methods and drawing from standardized procedures, the ambition is that guideline developers can evaluate the benefits, harms and costs of interventions, and derive explicit estimates of the probability of each outcome from their detached, objective stance.

This approach to evidence-based practice has been embraced by some within the social work profession, while others question the applicability of a scientific model for social work. Evidence-based practice in social work is being shaped to meet the nature and demands of the profession. While the scientific, 'gold standard' approach has been influential, there are other paradigms that are also shaping evidence-based practice in social work. An orientation towards critical self-evaluation, practical applications, client empowerment and accepting different interpretations of experience is influencing the development of evidence-based social work. The emerging identity of evidence-based social work is the focus of the next chapter.

Systematic review work is discussed in this chapter in respect of its centrality in defining formalized knowledge within a discipline or area of clinical practice. The method of systematic review is intended to appraise and synthesize evidence on social and behavioural interventions and public policy, including education, criminal justice and social work. The main purpose of systematic review work is shown to be in examining the effectiveness of intervention programs in affecting behaviour and in exploring whether there is evidence to suggest that particular intervention strategies have been effective in the settings in which they have been tried. It involves standardized procedures that identify criteria for the inclusion of studies, search strategies for study identification, data management and extraction indices, criteria for evaluating eligibility of studies, and analysis of variance statistical procedures. Characteristics for the exclusion of research studies include factors such as 'not a randomized controlled trial' or 'no other treatment controls involved'. While the primary concern is with evidence about the effectiveness of interventions and policies, effectiveness is influenced by variations in process and implementation, intervention components and recipients, as well as other factors.

At its pinnacle, the expectation of a systematic review is to define a focus for a practitioner audience for the guideline; to retrieve, evaluate and synthesize the evidence; to determine the appropriateness of the intervention; and to summarize their benefits and harms. Here we provide two representative case study examples of how this is constructed for particular interventions in child abuse and domestic violence scenarios. We show how cognitive-behavioural intervention has come to dominate as a preferred model by focusing on (i) 'cognitive-behavioural interventions for children who have been sexually abused' by Macdonald *et al.*

(2006); and (ii) 'cognitive behavioural therapy for violent men who batter female partners' by Smedslund *et al.* (2007). We discuss the various shortcomings of this systematic review work in terms of providing guidance to policy and practice interventions.

The next phase of the cycle is then discussed as we consider the link between research and practice. Evidence-based practice is framed in policy and best practice guidelines and is intended for implementation in practice settings. We examine literature on implementation and describe various strategies for the implementation of evidence-based practice in social work.

The hierarchy of evidence

A hierarchy that establishes the relative scientific quality of evidence is one of the hallmarks of medical evidence-based practice. The hierarchy and levels of evidence are well established and institutionalized in the work of the Cochrane Collaboration (Cochrane Collaboration nd: 1; Upshur *et al.* 2001). The Campbell Collaboration has sought to replicate the medical evidence standards of the Cochrane Collaboration in the social science fields of education, criminology and social welfare but has struggled to gain the same momentum, support and productivity of its sister network (Campbell Collaboration, nd). This hierarchical approach to evidence has also attracted a following within the social work profession (Gambrill 1999, 2006a; Gibbs and Gambrill 2002; Macdonald 2001; Macdonald and Sheldon 1992; Reid 2001; Sheldon 1986; Soydan 2008; Thyer 2002, 2006). A review of the levels of evidence in the hierarchy is offered here, with particular attention paid to how the different types of evidence are relevant to understanding the effectiveness of social interventions.

Randomized controlled trials

At the top of the evidence hierarchy sits the esteemed randomized controlled trial (RCT). RCTs are experimental studies designed to measure the effects of an intervention and are regarded as providing the strongest evidence about causal links between intervention and outcomes. So strong is the status of the RCT that there has been deliberation within the Cochrane and Campbell Collaborations about whether anything else really counts as evidence for effectiveness, and many reviews include only RCT studies (Shadish and Myers 2004). Generally RCTs involve the random allocation of clients to intervention (treatment) and control (non-treatment) groups. The Cochrane Collaboration defines an RCT as follows:

> An experiment in which two or more interventions, possibly including a control intervention or no intervention, are compared by being randomly allocated to participants. In most trials, an intervention is assigned to each individual, but sometimes assignment is to defined groups of individuals (for example in a household).
>
> (Cochrane Collaboration nd: 2)

Mirroring the Cochrane Collaboration, the Campbell Collaboration has also embraced randomized field trials (RFTs) as the community-based equivalent to the clinical RCT. Using the same experimental model, individuals, organizations or entire communities are randomly assigned to one of two or more intervention programs.

The purpose of the randomized experimental design is to determine the outcomes of the intervention/s, through measurement of group characteristics before and after the intervention and then comparing the experimental group to a control group. Despite the enthusiasm about what RCTs can offer, predictions by proponents that randomized social experiments will shape effectiveness research and guide social interventions in the future have not been achieved to the extent that was expected (Boruch 1994).

The RCT has strong internal validity. That is, it can be said with a high degree of certainty that in this setting, this particular intervention resulted in these outcomes for these particular people. If, however, these results are to be generalized to other settings and other people, then additional requirements must be placed on the RCT. Large, and randomly selected, representative samples are required in order to generalize findings to a wider population beyond the experimental groups. For social work interventions, attention would need to be paid to the range of variables in individuals, organizational settings and socio-cultural contexts that could impact upon the intervention outcome. These variables ideally would be controlled in the clinical experiment or field trial. This would warrant an even larger sample, often unrealistic for the types of interventions and contexts with which social workers engage in practice. By controlling these variables, the experiment is able to identify whether there is a causal link between the intervention and the outcome. The challenge often raised against the RCT in relation to social research is that the controlled conditions imposed by the experimental design oversimplify causal relationships and hence do not reflect the multi-dimensional and multi-directional nature of causation in the social world.

The RCT and RFT require that the intervention is well defined, standardized and replicable. Exactly the same intervention must be administered in the same way to every participant in the experimental group. This is another challenge for social work research, as interventions are intrinsically associated with, and vary according to, the individual skills and style of the social worker as well as the history and dynamics of the organizational context.

Another important limitation of the RCT for social intervention research is that the desirable outcomes of the intervention must be measurable. Despite the existence of banks of psychometric tests, the validity of measures of many social, emotional and human characteristics remains open to interpretation and dispute. Not only must outcomes be measurable, but there also needs to be agreement on what the desired outcomes of the intervention actually are. A well-designed RCT may produce strong evidence for a causal relationship between intervention and outcome, but there could be disagreement about whether this outcome is actually the desirable one. An outcome may be assessed not because it is the most desirable outcome, but because it is a measurable outcome. Drawing on an example from a medical review, when treatments are given to address the effects of sleep deprivation, outcomes in terms of cardiovascular health are not of direct relevance but findings about this may still colour perceptions of the treatment and its effectiveness (Stradling and Davies 1997). Multiple outcomes can be assessed by RCTs but, again, these must be defined, delineated and measurable.

Medical treatments may lend themselves more readily to this type of experimental assessment of effectiveness than do social interventions, given the comparative ability to standardize medical treatments and treatment conditions. But even within medicine, concerns about the limitations of evidence from RCTs are being expressed (Blau 1997; Charlton 1997; Morgan 1997; Stradling and Davies 1997). In attempts to replicate the 'gold standard' of RCTs in social intervention research, the focus of attention has been skewed toward promoting internal validity of experiments to the detriment of external validity. This is a concerning development when the purpose of evidence-based practice, it would seem, is to generate evidence that has external validity. That is, evidence that can be used to inform real interventions, by real practitioners in real contexts with all their complexities and individual differences. The implications of trading external validity for internal validity are pointed out by Kenneth Howe (2004: 45):

> Putting a premium on internal validity encourages educational researchers to focus on easy-to-manipulate, simplistic interventions and to avoid questions about existing policy and practice that for one reason or another, are not suited to being investigated via randomized experiments.

The oversimplification of causal relationships and limits on how far results can be generalized, as outlined above, are reasons why RCTs may be passed over as a method for social research. The requirement that standardized, replicable interventions are applied is also a limiting factor in designing RCT studies of social work interventions. From the 'gold standard', scientific perspective, however, the RCT would only be regarded as inappropriate if there were ethical concerns or logistical limitations. This may include ethical concerns about withholding treatment or potentially beneficial programs from control group participants or practical concerns relating to the potential to recruit sufficient participants and gain the cross-section of participants required to control for interfering variables. Proponents of the RCT and RFT models argue that, given the strength of the results that experimental designs can yield, there is an imperative for social researchers to work on overcoming the difficulties and addressing the limitations, rather than discarding the model. Thomas Cook and Monique Payne (2002) carefully consider a list of common objections to RFT educational research and offer ways to conceptualize and manage experimental research that address these objections. Likewise, Gibbs and Gambrill (2002) dissect the objections in the context of social work research. The limitations of the RCT and RFT have, nonetheless, brought into question whether this type of evaluation research can be held up as the 'gold standard' for educational, social work and other social intervention research in the same way that it is in the medical sciences. Cook and Payne (2002: 174), while remaining strong advocates of experimental design, think not:

In some quarters, particularly medical ones, the randomized experiment is considered the causal 'gold standard'. It is clearly not that in educational contexts, given the difficulties with implementing and maintaining randomly created groups ...

It may not be possible to achieve all the conditions for definitive answers to practice questions in a single experimental study, and this is why the evidence-based practice approach does not rely on the findings of a single study. It is the accumulation and appraisal of research findings over time that contribute to judgements about best evidence. This is where a distinction between efficacy and effectiveness is usefully drawn. Efficacy, or positive outcomes, of social work interventions determined in well-controlled experimental research designs suggests that while confined by the specific testing environment, the intervention is promising (Soydan 2008). Effectiveness studies can then be conducted in a variety of less controlled but real life conditions to examine outcomes. Effectiveness research determines the diverse conditions in which interventions work and the extent of their success in achieving positive change.

Quasi-experimental studies

Quasi-experimental designs have been used as a way of dealing with some of the ethical, resource and practical concerns associated with RCTs. For the proponents of scientific, 'gold standard' evidence, quasi-experiments sit on the tier below the RCT on the hierarchy of evidence. Quasi-experimental design has the same structure as the RCT, but does not entail random allocation of interventions to participants. It relies, rather, on using naturally occurring or convenient groups to undertake treatment or control interventions (e.g., using people on the waiting list as the control group). In order to compare the groups, participants in the intervention and non-intervention groups are required to be matched according to relevant criteria. Without randomization, selection biases are likely to impact upon the findings of quasi-experimental studies. A still weaker quasi-experimental design involves the comparison of the same group before and after an intervention, without a control group. Causal relationships cannot, however, be determined from this design.

Single-case (single-system or time-series) designs

The single-case research design entails multiple testing of a particular characteristic or characteristics among a group of study participants to establish a baseline measure prior to the intervention. Multiple testing occurs again after the intervention, allowing for a comparison before and after the intervention. This is a stronger design than the simple pre- and post-test, as the multiple testing reduces the impact of interfering variables. The benefit of this design is that it can yield results about causation from a small sample of participants. A drawback includes the limited ability to generalize beyond the sample, unless a large, representative sample is recruited. Another concern with the single-case design is the intrusive nature of multiple testings, particularly for vulnerable clients, and the potential for these testings to affect the impact of the intervention. During the empirical clinical practice movement of the 1970s and 1980s, the single-case design was heralded as a research design particularly suited to the needs of social work evaluation studies and it continues to be a method successfully applied to the evaluation of social work services (Thyer and Kazi 2004). The single 'case' under study may be an individual, a family, a group, an organization or a community.

As for RCT designs, the quasi-experimental designs including single-case rely upon the use of standardized interventions and the measurement of specific, defined desirable outcomes. This limits applicability to much social work practice.

Cohort studies

A cohort study involves the observation over a period of time of a group of people who have had a particular experience that equates with an intervention (e.g., children who have been in foster care). Subsets of the group may be compared (e.g., those placed in foster care with siblings and those placed without siblings) or the group may be compared with a control group, to strengthen findings about relationships (i.e., children who have not been in foster care). The cohort study generates weaker evidence than the RCT, as the intervention (foster care) cannot be randomly allocated to the study participants. Random selection of large samples from the population groups (children in foster care and children not in foster care) will, however, strengthen the external validity, i.e., the ability to make generalizations about the population groups or subgroups.

Case control studies

Case control studies are similar to cohort studies in that they track a group of people over time. The main difference is that selection of participants for the case control study is on the basis of an outcome characteristic, rather than an intervention or experience. Cases that have the particular outcome characteristic are then compared to a control group that does not have this characteristic. The information on the two groups is gathered, either prospectively or retrospectively, in order to find associations between the outcome characteristic and exposure to particular experiences, interventions or risk factors. An example of a case control study would be the comparison between a group of women who suffer from depression and a group of women without depression in terms of experiences of violence throughout their lives. A weakness of this design, in terms of the strength of the evidence, is that interventions (violence) are not under the control of the researchers and hence cannot be administered in standardized and measurable ways. This, of course, would not be desirable, which is why certain social issues are appropriately addressed by this study design. Again, the external validity of the study (ability to generalize) would be strengthened by random selection of large samples from the case population (women who experience depression) and the control population (women without depression).

Qualitative studies

Qualitative research encompasses a variety of methods and theoretical approaches. Grounded theory, narrative, phenomenology and action research are qualitative research approaches that have gained recognition in social work. Qualitative studies can be used to gather detailed information on experiences and meanings associated with interventions through, for example, observation, interviews, focus groups and analysis of existing transcript data such as case files. A qualitative research approach examines the complex and multi-dimensional nature of human experience and seeks to gather information on the range of circumstances and factors that impact on this experience. Themes, patterns and trends are identified, but attention is also paid to explanations of experiences that fall outside the dominant patterns. A qualitative research design allows researchers to engage with participants in a holistic and meaningful way about their experiences of a particular intervention and its effectiveness. This is in contrast to an experimental approach, which entails reducing multi-dimensional people to quantifiable variables that can be measured.

Within the scientific paradigm that strives for 'gold standard' evidence, qualitative research may be undertaken because ethical or logistical concerns place limits on experimental research. Qualitative studies are regarded, at best, as an adjunct to experimental research and traditionally sit at the bottom of the evidence hierarchy as a 'weak' form of evidence. The absence of controls and strict measurement in qualitative research are regarded as features of poor design that will not allow causal links between intervention and outcome to be determined as they can be in experimental studies. Qualitative studies tend to focus on small samples or particular contexts, which does not allow results to be directly generalized. The benefit of a qualitative approach, however, is that the characteristics of the particular sample, context and intervention can be described in some detail so that decisions about applicability to other settings can be made by readers in an informed way. The Cochrane Collaboration is beginning to pay attention to qualitative research as evidence in healthcare and has developed a qualitative methods group to advise on and facilitate the inclusion of qualitative evidence in medical reviews of effectiveness (Cochrane Collaboration nd: 3).

Practice wisdom and expert opinion

Social workers draw on more than research findings to provide evidence for their practices. They draw on a 'complex mix of moral, rational and pragmatic reasons' to justify interventions (Colgan and Cheers 2002: 115) and a variety of practice-based 'evidence' in complex and ambiguous ways (Shaw and Shaw 1997). Using this type of practice wisdom as evidence has drawn criticism within the evidence-based practice movement as a strategy used to uphold accepted practices in an uncritical and authoritative way (Gambrill 1999, 2004; Thyer and Kazi 2004). It is open to debate as to whether practice wisdom can be regarded as a source of evidence or whether practice competence exists in another realm that can be augmented by evidence. Gambrill (2006a) does, however, list expert opinion as a source of evidence, albeit level five in a hierarchy with five levels. She describes expert opinion as the consensual agreement among 'experts' located in research-based centres, which is different from the practice wisdom developed by individual social workers or within local teams. In the medical context, there are dangers in ignoring practitioners' clinical knowledge about the appropriate practice questions to ask and relevant clinical factors to include in studies (Blau 1997; Charlton 1997; Morgan 1997; Stradling and Davies 1997).

Debating the hierarchy

Given the limitations of experimental designs for understanding the complex issues surrounding intervention effectiveness in social work, as outlined above, it is important that evidence about causal links under experimental conditions be viewed critically. Why the identification of a narrowly defined causal relationship should be regarded as more valuable evidence than detailed qualitative information on the experiences of social work effectiveness is an issue of debate. While experimental research can be appropriate to investigate certain impacts of social work interventions, it is the privilege given to the dominant paradigm, associated techniques and research language that is questioned in regard to the particular issues confronted in social work effectiveness research. If experimental research produces reliable information about unrealistically defined constructs in controlled circumstances, the wider applicability and usefulness for social work is limited. In comparison to some medical interventions, social work effectiveness research presents particular problems around standardizing interventions, randomization and external validity. These are not, however, peculiarly social work concerns. The usefulness of qualitative inquiry, over experimental designs, to understanding the nature, quality and context of interventions has been revealed in public health, community health and medicine (Hausman 2002; Malterud 2001; Warburton and Black 2002) and in educational research (Cannella and Lincoln 2004; Howe 2004).

Qualitative research, like experimental research, has its limitations. Qualitative research, however, offers a different type of evidence to that generated by experimental approaches. Qualitative research can offer information to help us understand the importance and relevance of interventions in people's lives (Shaw 1999). The features of social work practice, how it works, for whom and why, standards of practice, how practice varies between practitioners and cultural or organizational context are issues that are suited to qualitative inquiry. Qualitative studies can provide useful findings that either stand alone or enhance and explain the findings of experimental studies. Findings from qualitative research can be used to develop and test theories and to better understand the nature and characteristics of complex phenomena, such as family dynamics. Apart from claims about the strength or weakness of different research designs, there are important questions to be asked about the appropriateness of research designs in providing findings that will inform real practice questions.

The complementary nature of qualitative and experimental research has been widely recognized in social work, where there is a growing emphasis on mixed-method approaches (Cheetham 1992, 1997; Gibbs 2001; Reid 2001; Shaw 1999, 2003; Sheldon 1986). Cheetham (1992), for example, claims that there is little point to studying the outcomes and effectiveness of social work interventions unless we also understand the processes involved in these interventions. Beyond social work, mixed-method approaches that bridge the divide between experimental and interpretive methodologies in social research are gaining prominence (Bergman 2008; Maxwell 2004; Plano Clark and Creswell 2007; Teddlie and Tashakkori 2008).

Rather than viewing evidence as a hierarchy determined by research methodology, evidence for effectiveness could more productively be viewed as a culmination of findings from a balanced combination of research methods and a variety of perspectives. This is more likely to offer useful knowledge about the impact of complex and varied social work practices than a preoccupation with the superiority of RCTs. Webb (2001) draws a useful distinction between evidence to determine and evidence to support. It is possible to determine the answers to some social work questions through experimental studies. But social workers, more often, are faced with practice questions for particular contexts and situations where there are no definitive answers. What is needed is a varied range of information that can support and justify decision-making in practice. Reductionist approaches to evidence-based practice are less likely to yield useful guidance for social workers than does a broad view of evidence for practice.

This view on the nature of evidence for social work is not, however, a generally accepted one in the realm of evidence-based practice. Reid (2001: 277), for example, puts forward the position that while qualitative methods can enrich understanding, they cannot be used to validate effectiveness and that 'scientific knowledge is the place to look when one is searching for definitive answers to questions about phenomena, whether physical or psychosocial'. Howe (2004) refers to such a stance as 'mixed-methods experimentalism', where qualitative approaches are recognized, but only as an inferior adjunct to experimentalism. This denies the important developments and applications of qualitative methodologies and the contributions that qualitative, interpretive inquiry has made to social research. Howe (2004) proposes that a shift in understanding of a mixed-method approach is required and argues for 'mixed-methods interpretivism' which acknowledges that the 'insider story' about meanings and experiences is fundamental to answering questions about causal relationships. This offers a democratic and inclusive balance to the technocratic emphasis in experimental designs. The distinction drawn is not in terms of methodology, but rather in terms of a preparedness to include the political and nuanced aspects of social life in research inquiry.

Gathering and critically reviewing a range of information that is used to guide social work practice decision-making is undoubtedly an important process in quality practice. The evidence-based practice movement has, however, created and institutionalized notions of good and bad evidence in this decision-making process. Quality evidence has become associated with scientific approaches, alienating research terminology and the capacities of research experts. The experimental designs are, however, limited in many ways, particularly for questions about social work interventions. The so-called 'gold standard' approach can produce results about narrow aspects of social work that may not be very useful for social workers grappling with the challenges of daily practice. While particular research techniques and standardized practices are employed in a 'gold standard' approach, the claim that these are more 'scientific' in the face of the various limitations of experimental design is open to question (Charlton 1997; Morgan 1997).

Social workers are continually required to respond creatively and reflectively to practice situations for which no definitive evidence about effectiveness is available. The evidence generated by 'the experts' takes on a status of authority, legitimacy and fact, when the research findings may actually be limited by research design and the value-laden cultural context in which the findings have been generated (Gibbs 2001; Webb 2001). The 'hard' facts generated by 'gold standard' RCTs can be useful as one source of information that contributes, along with other evidence, to a generally incomplete understanding of impact and effectiveness. Evidence for practice is also gained from the less tangible experiences, principles and processes that can be studied through well-constructed qualitative research and provide knowledge on causal relationships and effectiveness.

As the research experts generate the evidence and shape the best practice guidelines, the experiences of clients and the practice wisdom of social workers are being disregarded as poor evidence in the process. This alienation of social workers and clients from the evidence-generation process should be addressed not only because of the direct experience that both have regarding the impact and effectiveness of interventions, but also because these are the people who are expected to implement and receive the products of evidence-based practice guidelines. The methodological fundamentalism associated with experimental design contributes to an elite and narrow construction of what is deemed to be 'truth' in social research. This diverts critical debate about issues of values, perspectives, power, oppression, public responsibility and where resources are being directed (Cannella and Lincoln 2004).

The language of evidence, 'gold standards', hierarchies, strong and weak evidence, and causal relationships serves to promote the valuing of certain knowledge over other knowledge. Qualitative and experiential knowledge could be valued for what it contributes to practice and policy decision-making. Marginalization within the institutions that generate evidence, however, suggests that this interpretive information focusing on personal, interpersonal and contextual factors will be overshadowed by findings from experimental studies. There is privilege, authority and a resource base associated with the systematic review of experimental research findings, regardless of their real strength and applicability to policy and practice.

Systematic reviews

The influence of the experimental research evidence paradigm is enhanced by the practice of systematic reviews. Fundamental to the evidence-based practice approach is the accumulation and systematic review of research data on a particular condition, intervention or issue. Systematic reviews gained prominence in medicine with the emergence of the Cochrane Collaboration in the 1990s and have become established practice. The systematic review is essentially an analysis of all of the available evidence, and a judgement about the effectiveness or otherwise of a practice. Systematic reviews can entail a synthesis of a range of theoretical and research literature relating to a practice issue. This broad, encompassing approach to systematic reviews can be unwieldy and hence systematic reviews may be confined to research entailing a particular methodological approach, such as experimental designs, which allows for a meta-analysis of findings. Meta-analyses, which are discussed in more detail below, involve the quantitative integration of results of the research that has been reviewed (Soydan 2008).

The Cochrane and Campbell Collaborations adopt narrow methodological restrictions and require the meta-analysis of findings in their evidence-production tasks. In line with the hierarchical approach to understanding evidence, a rigorous, standardized but exclusive approach to research reviews has been implemented. The Cochrane and Campbell Collaborations have adopted standardized processes and techniques for searching, reviewing and reporting research literature that regard RCTs as the only really valuable evidence.

The rationale for conducting systematic reviews is that policy-makers and practitioners need a research base for decision-making, but are faced with competing claims made by researchers and advocacy groups. The systematic review aims to provide a standardized and unbiased appraisal of the accumulated body of evidence from multiple studies. A statistical combination of findings provides information on the effect of policies and programs that is regarded as more precise than what could be offered by a single study or by the synthesis of research findings from studies utilizing a range of theoretical and methodological approaches (Boruch *et al.* 2001).

Systematic reviews are conducted by teams of researchers over a substantial period of time. A systematic review for the Cochrane or Campbell Collaboration starts with the reviewers preparing a review protocol proposal. This proposal is expected to demonstrate scientific rigour and provide a plan for periodic updating. It is subjected to peer review prior to implementation. The protocol is required to address the following (Boruch *et al.* 2001):

1 *Questions or hypotheses which will be pursued in the review.* Questions should be specific regarding the participants, setting, interventions and outcomes to be investigated.
2 *Criteria that will be used to select the literature.* The inclusion criteria should address the participants of the primary studies, the intervention and the outcomes. In addition, they should also specify what research methodologies will be considered for inclusion in the review, e.g., RCTs, quasi-experiments, case studies, and so on.
3 *Strategy that will be used to identify all relevant literature within an agreed time frame.* This should include electronic databases and bibliographies that will be searched, and the search terms that will be used. Both published

and unpublished studies in all languages are to be sought. The Campbell Collaboration has established a register of controlled trials as a resource in the searching process (C2-SPECTUR).

4 *A study selection process.* Eligibility of studies should be independently assessed by more than one reviewer and a strategy is required to review any disagreements. A record of excluded studies and reasons for exclusions should be kept.

5 *Guideline for how the quality of primary studies will be assessed or critically appraised and any exclusion criteria based on quality considerations.* Assessments are made of the strength, validity and quality of studies through examination of how attrition of participants is handled, sampling and randomization.

6 *Details on how data will be extracted from the primary research regarding the participants, the intervention, the outcome measures, and the results.* A data extraction form is developed and, ideally, reviewers should be blinded to information about the study authors, institutions and journals.

7 *A plan of how the extracted data will be pooled.* Statistical analysis – meta-analysis – may or may not be used in pooling numerical data from findings of the studies included in the review. This will depend on the nature and quality of studies. Where possible, odds ratio (for categorical outcome data) or standardized mean differences (for continuous data) and their 95 per cent confidence intervals are calculated for each included study. If appropriate with available data, results from comparable groups of studies are then pooled with statistical meta-analysis using Review Manager software from the Cochrane Collaboration, which also tests the heterogeneity between the combined results using a standard chi-square test. For textual data, the current convention is to develop a narrative summary. With the emergence of the Qualitative Assessment and Review Instrument (QARI), it is anticipated that textual analysis – meta-synthesis – will become the convention in reviews of this nature. While it may not be possible to state exactly what analysis will be undertaken, the general approach should be included in the protocol.

On completion of the review, reviewers are required to interpret the results in terms of strength of findings, limitations, statistical power, applicability to clinical practice, economic implications and implications for future research.

Case examples

In order to illustrate the systematic review process, what it has to offer and its limitations, two case examples will be presented. These two reviews are registered with both the Campbell and Cochrane Collaborations.

1 'Cognitive-behavioural interventions for children who have been sexually abused' by Macdonald *et al.* (2006).

  The purpose of this review is stated as being 'to assess the efficacy of cognitive-behavioural approaches (CBT) in addressing the immediate and longer-term sequelae on children who have been sexually abused' (Macdonald *et al.* 2006: 3). Part of the rationale for the focus of the review is that CBT has a promising record of evidence in dealing with a range of problems and that previous reviews in this area have suggested that CBT is effective. So here we have an example of evidence building on evidence, but without a convincing rationale for why CBT was chosen to review over another type of intervention. As more research and more reviews of research are done on a particular type of intervention, such as CBT, this can become established as the intervention of choice to implement and evaluate. In the review process there is incidental regard given to other interventions that may be working effectively but may not have been researched, or not researched in the right way (RCTs) in order to warrant a systematic review. The systematic review thus can be a way of enhancing and reinforcing intervention fads with disregard for other interventions that may be equally effective.

The types of studies included in the review are experimental designs that entailed random or quasi-random allocation to experimental and control groups. The participants in all studies were children up to eighteen years of age who have experienced sexual assault. It is recognized by the reviewers that CBT encompasses a range of intervention styles and types and hence they rely on the description of the intervention as CBT by the authors of the studies. The interventions varied in terms of number and length of sessions, whether or not parents were included and whether individual or group therapy was provided. The style and skill of particular practitioners would further impact on the variation in the nature of the interventions under study. Only studies that evaluated effectiveness in terms of standardized, peer-reviewed, psychometric outcome measures (e.g., of depression, anxiety and sexualized behaviour) were included in the review.

The reviewers list in detail the databases and key words that were used to search for relevant studies: 377 records were identified from the search and, of these, ten studies (twelve papers) were assessed as meeting the criteria summarized above and hence were included in the review; 365 research studies were excluded from the review. All qualitative research was excluded as well as quantitative-experimental studies that did not meet the minimum criteria for a well-planned and implemented design. Such is the faith put in the value of randomized experimental designs that the vast majority of studies were excluded. In this review, reliance is placed upon specified research techniques and narrow outcome measures.

The selected ten studies, however, by no means offered the strong experimental evidence promoted as the 'gold standard'. The varied nature of the interventions under study makes it difficult to draw conclusions about what is effective. Attrition rates in all studies were high and inadequately explained. There were potential biases in most studies, with researchers knowing which participants were from the experimental groups and which were from the control groups. The reviewers state that the quality aspects of the studies were poorly reported, that there are a range of methodological weaknesses and that the quality of evidence is poor. The meta-analysis of data from these poor experimental studies found some small positive effects, but these were mostly not significant. The authors conclude that 'There is nothing in this review to detract from the general consensus that cognitive-behavioural approaches ... merit consideration as a treatment of choice for sexually abused children ...' (Macdonald *et al.* 2006: 9) and that more and better experimental research should be conducted.

While this statement may offer encouragement for those engaged in CBT work, the findings are of no use to someone wishing to make a critical and informed choice about the appropriateness of CBT over other types of interventions. A practitioner who is questioning the domination of CBT over other types of responses to child sexual assault – including more comprehensive educational, psychological and community-based interventions – is faced with a statement about 'general consensus' and 'merit' that is not actually based in evidence, but carries the weight and influence of a Cochrane Review. There are risks associated with reporting inconclusive findings from systematic reviews. Funding may be withdrawn from services supporting children who have been sexually abused if there is no evidence to support effectiveness. It is, therefore, understandable that Macdonald *et al.* (2006) have phrased their conclusions in the way that they have. The implications of doing this, however, is that support for more comprehensive, far-reaching and costly interventions than CBT could suffer as a consequence. While CBT may be effective, it is not the answer to social problems. It is a relatively standardized, psychological intervention that lends itself nicely to experimental study. It is a current fad that is generating research and reviews that further substantiate its domination. CBT is a contained, individualized intervention that does not address the complex issues surrounding gender-based violence at community and social levels. The data gathered in the 365 studies excluded from the review may shed some light on some of the issues around implementing CBT, its strengths and limitations. These studies may not determine relationships between intervention and outcome, but nor do the studies in this review. While Macdonald *et al.* (2006) recommend more and better RCTs to address this, perhaps, at this time, we need to better understand the range of interventions. What are children's experiences of the interventions? Why are people not continuing with therapy (explaining high attrition rates in RCTs)? What are children, parents and therapists expecting and getting from the interventions (these may not match with the psychometric measures needed for RCTs)? What aspects of the interventions work well from the perspectives of participants and what aspects do not? What have been different experiences in different contexts? These are all useful questions for practitioners to ask and a range of research findings may help practitioners to formulate informed judgements about these questions. This systematic review, however, does not. A CBT therapist, with an uncritical approach to practice may, however, be buoyed by the conclusions.

2 'Cognitive behavioural therapy for violent men who batter female partners'
by Smedslund *et al.* (2007).

Another example of the current interest in gathering evidence for, and
hence promoting, the profile of CBT is the systematic review by Smedslund
et al. (2007: 3) which aims 'to measure the effects of cognitive behaviour
therapy (CBT) and similar interventions on men's physical abuse of their
female partners'. The review included only RCTs and quasi-experiments. The
control groups varied and included waiting list, no intervention or another
intervention. Similar to the Macdonald *et al.* (2006) review, the intervention
included a range of treatments (individual, couple or group treatment in a
variety of settings). If the study authors identified the treatment as CBT or
the treatment was 'recognizably so', then the studies were included in the
review. Experimental designs are thus limited, given that the treatment is not
standardized and reproducible.

The outcome of interest in the review is the level of violent behaviour
toward female partners. This outcome is not reliant upon a psychometric scale,
but does depend upon access to reliable reporting mechanisms (self-reports,
victim reports, and court and police reports). As violent behaviour includes
verbal aggression and hostile attitudes, outcomes were somewhat open to
interpretation.

Database searching and study review techniques have been carefully
described in the review with a level of detail that would allow the process to
be replicated. The results of the search produced 1,969 records of which 1,724
were 'clearly irrelevant'; 245 studies remained, of which 75 were selected for
closer examination. Reading these reports resulted in further studies being
discarded, leaving twelve studies that reported on six RCTs. It is hard to
believe that none of the enormous number of studies that were discarded by the
reviewers could offer useful knowledge on the effectiveness of interventions.
No doubt many of these studies were undertaken by reputable and skilled
researchers and while there may be inadequacies, or alternative methodologies,
so too are there limitations in the experimental designs selected for inclusion.
For the dozen studies included, there is a lack of standardization in regard to
both intervention and outcome measures. The reviewers conclude that the
methodological quality was low, that there was a high risk of bias for the studies
included and that the outcome measures are likely to have been affected by
support services to female partners who subsequently felt more able to report
abuse. High attrition rates for intervention programs are identified as a likely
contributor to bias in the study samples. Despite these concerns, these studies
have been selected for the review because they are controlled experimental
designs. Given the limitations in the studies selected for the review, it is not
surprising that the reviewers conclude that:

> ... research evidence is insufficient to draw conclusions about the effec-
> tiveness of cognitive behavioural interventions for spouse abusers in
> reducing or eliminating male violence against female partners. Note that

this does not mean that there is evidence for no effect.

(Smedslund *et al.* 2007: 8)

What is surprising is the conclusion that 'there is a need for more, and larger-scale, randomised interventions' (*ibid.*: 8). How can this be concluded when there is so much research in the field that has not been reviewed? There is no acknowledgement that the RCT method of research may not suit the nature of the therapeutic interventions, the nature of the client group and the social and interpersonal context in which outcomes must be assessed. Even if interventions were to be standardized, a lack of compliance with treatment and hence high attrition rates are likely to remain a feature. It would also be unethical to withhold support to female partners in order to control variables impacting upon reporting rates. Factors in the criminal justice system will continue to impact upon who is directed toward treatment and who is diverted. But rather than a critical appraisal of these contextual factors and informed decision-making about appropriate methods for investigation, the RCT is unquestionably accepted as what is needed in order to identify evidence for CBT. The unconvincing reason that the authors give for this is that it 'has been possible in other fields, such as welfare to work ...' (Smedslund *et al.* 2007: 8). Perhaps the RCT is an appropriate methodology to investigate some other social intervention questions, but it faces considerable barriers in regard to the practice question for this review.

Critiquing the systematic review: does it work?

Essentially, the expectation of a systematic review is to:

1 define a focus for a practitioner audience for the guideline in terms of intervention and population group;
2 retrieve, evaluate and synthesize the evidence;
3 determine the appropriateness of the intervention;
4 summarize the benefits or harms.

The standardization of techniques associated with the systematic review process is aimed at producing an unbiased, objective and rigorous process. In line with principles around adopting a hierarchy of evidence, the systematic review assumes that scientific principles and rules are superior to interpretation and judgement. The review process relies upon a clear statement of relevance criteria, an explicit hierarchy of research designs (acceptable and unacceptable evidence), a well-described process that is replicable and minimal discretion. The tension between the scientific paradigm and interpretive judgement has, however, resulted in debate about the usefulness of the systematic review. What is missing from the systematic review is exactly what it seeks to avoid – reviewer judgement. Hammersley (2001: 548) advocates for a narrative approach to the review of research that incorporates reviewer judgement:

> Producing a review of the literature is a distinctive task in its own right. It is not a matter of 'synthesising data' … It can involve judgement on the validity of the findings and conclusions of particular studies and thinking about how these relate to one another, and how their interrelations can be used to illuminate the field under investigation. This will require the reviewer to draw on his or her tacit knowledge, derived from experience, and to think about the substantive and methodological issues, not just to apply replicable procedures.

The effect of a standardized, technical approach to the systematic review is, like the hierarchy of evidence, privileging a particular type of research that is narrowly focused around measurable interventions and outcomes. Again, the concern is that qualitative, interpretive and participatory research findings are overlooked in decisions about policy and practice responses to social issues.

The two reviews examined above do not offer any guidance for the practitioner or policy-maker seeking evidence to inform decision-making about where to direct time and energy so that the most effective outcomes are achieved. But how representative are these two reviews of the systematic review work undertaken by the Campbell Collaboration? The Campbell Collaboration was inaugurated in 2000 with a plan to provide resources for decision-making in the social welfare, criminal justice and educational fields through systematically reviewing and disseminating research findings from high-quality research studies (Boruch *et al.* 2001). There are three active groups within the collaboration. The Social Welfare Group has fallen short of its original goal of five to ten reviews per year, with twenty-one completed reviews available in the library (Campbell Collaboration n.d.). While a few of these reviews concluded *some* evidence for effectiveness of the interventions under investigation, this is generally guarded and most reviews are inconclusive due to insufficient evidence. The number of reviews produced by the Education Group has been even more disappointing, with the five published reviews falling far short of the ten to fifteen anticipated reviews per annum. The Crime and Justice Group has produced fourteen reviews, whereas thirty reviews were anticipated in three years. The small number of reviews and the extremely limited usefulness of these reviews for practice must bring into question the appropriateness of this approach to evidence generation for areas of practice such as social work.

It is apparent from the titles of reviews that research studies investigating discrete and standardized interventions are being favoured in the review process. This is understandable, as it is these types of interventions that lend themselves to evaluation by experimental designs. But as discussed above, even the more standardized interventions, such as CBT, are varied in nature and pose limitations on what can be concluded from a meta-analysis of experimental studies. Cognitive behavioural approaches derive theoretically and empirically from four theories of learning: respondent conditioning (associative learning), operant conditioning (the effect of the environment on patterns of behaviour, particularly reinforcement and punishment), observational learning (learning by imitation) and cognitive learning (the impact of thought patterns on feelings and behaviour) (Macdonald *et al.* 2006). These more standardized interventions are, however, only a small part of the range of complex social interventions. The systematic review process is raising the profile of certain interventions, but this could have a detrimental effect on the recognition of other interventions that may be equally effective.

Meta-analysis for research synthesis

While we have indicated the importance of meta-analysis in relation to systematic reviews in discussing the Campbell and Cochrane Collaboration approaches above, it is also important to recognize that the meta-analysis does not offer a means to incorporate research using the range of methodological and theoretical approaches. Research findings do not always lend themselves to the quantitative synthesis required in a meta-analysis, and in these situations alternative approaches to research synthesis are needed. Meta-analysis together with experimental design have, however, achieved a rising status in the field of evidence-based practice which has overshadowed this more encompassing approach to systematic review and research synthesis.

The purpose of the meta-analysis is to consolidate findings from a range of empirical studies investigating the same research hypothesis (or practice question). Meta-analysis is 'a specific statistical strategy for assembling the results of several studies into a single estimate' (Sackett *et al*. 1996: 4). When some studies have small sample sizes, the meta-analysis can be an effective way to increase the statistical power of findings about the effect of interventions. Drawing on a range of studies conducted in different settings will also strengthen conclusions about the reliability of interventions across different practice contexts. The quality of the meta-analysis, however, is reliant upon the methodological quality and measurement standardization across the studies included. The synthesis of findings for the meta-analysis has the potential to conceal methodological inadequacies and inconsistencies. Publication bias could also be an issue if only published studies were incorporated into the meta-analysis, when studies that found no effect were less likely to have been published. The conclusions drawn from meta-analyses do need to be viewed critically and, while offering a way to synthesize findings, the meta-analysis limits the scope of a systematic review of literature. The response of some social work commentators to such concerns has been a push to strengthen the methodological rigour of both the primary studies and the meta-analysis techniques (Littell 2005; Littell *et al*. 2008). In order for the findings of a meta-analysis to be useful as evidence for practice, however, it would seem that both the methodological and contextual details of the included studies should be examined in depth. A process of informed interpretation is required, in conjunction with methodological rigour, to identify not only the interventions that are effective but also the principles of practice that are associated with effectiveness (Lipsey 2003, 2009). A meta-analysis that relies on a high level of scientific rigour will still have a narrow focus and is unable to incorporate insights derived from theoretical or qualitative enquiries (Lipsey and Wilson 2000).

Evidence for practice: the challenges of implementation

This chapter has offered a critical appraisal of the hierarchical approach to evidence, experimental design, the systematic review and meta-analysis. A review of two case examples of systematic reviews and an overview of the work of the Campbell Collaboration as it relates to social work does not offer an encouraging picture. Social work advocates for 'gold standard' evidence are faced with challenging questions about whether this approach can fulfil expectations of strong, definitive answers about causal relationships or if it is missing vital and useful information about impact and effectiveness by focusing on a definition of evidence that is too narrow and a research methodology that does not match with the realities of the real world and human behaviour. Will an insistence on 'gold standard' evidence result in the production of useful evidence that will inform practitioners and policy-makers as they make difficult decisions about interventions and resource distribution, or does it serve only to legitimate certain practices through technical processes, institutional cultures and financial support? The evidence-based practice movement claims to challenge the uncritical acceptance of authority and standard practices, by being anti-authoritarian, rigorous and scientific (Gambrill 1999; Thyer and Kazi 2004). The 'gold standard' approach to evidence-based practice appears, however, to be doing the opposite. Standard, technical procedures are employed, rather than critical analysis and informed judgements. The experimental design is upheld despite contextual factors that threaten the ability to apply the model in the controlled way that will produce strong evidence. Technical and alienating language is adopted by the expert authority and used to legitimize certain interventions over others when 'evidence' is slim and unconvincing.

We discuss the specific factors relating to the implementation of evidence-based social work in Chapter 6. However, we may ask at this juncture whether evidence-based practice can be implemented in social work practice and, if so, what the required strategies and processes are that will move beyond the current work of the Campbell Collaboration to a situation that more adequately meets the needs of policy-makers and practitioners. Mullen (2006) outlines the challenges that need to be faced in conducting systematic reviews of research for social work practice. He provides a list of questions relating to outcome measures that require resolution if the systematic review were to produce information on outcomes that could be applied in practice. Social workers are concerned with intervention outcomes that are complex, diverse and change over time. A systematic review of research should approach the evaluation of outcomes as if such results were to be meaningful for those in practice. While Mullen's list of questions for resolution is daunting, and would likely be a deterrent for diligent researchers, it does provide a framework for approaching the range of factors that require consideration in producing evidence that is not only strong but also useful and applicable for social work. The 'Guidelines for dementia care' developed by the Social Care Institute of Excellence (SCIE) in the UK is an example of practice guidelines that have taken an inclusive, non-hierarchical approach to evidence and have acknowledged the importance of practitioner expertise and judgements in practice (Gould and Kendall 2007).

Importantly, the guidelines are not seen as an end in themselves. Resources and support strategies have been put in place in acknowledgement of the fact that implementation will not be automatic, but needs to be a process that entails revising old practices and promoting new ones.

The production of applicable evidence is the start, but is not sufficient for implementation of evidence-based practice to occur. Mullen, Shlonsky *et al.* (2005) draw on a model by Haynes that presents clinical expertise as the focal point through which the practitioner integrates the assessment of evidence with assessments of both client preferences and the contextual circumstances in making practice decisions. A commitment of time, education and resources is required within the organization, however, to facilitate this integration of evidence at the level of practice. Mullen *et al.* (2007) identify five strategies to facilitate the movement from evidence dissemination to the implementation of evidence-based practice in social work. Essentially, these entail:

1 social work education that incorporates evidence-based practice as an integral component of professional training;
2 dissemination of practical resources and guidelines to assist practitioners in implementing practices that are well supported by evidence;
3 experts being available to consult with practitioners about practice questions;
4 developing evidence-based cultures in organizations through staff training and team development activities;
5 the social work profession setting goals and targets around achieving evidence-based practice outcomes in relation to research, training and development of organizational cultures.

Mullen *et al.* (2008) emphasize that these strategies must be tailored to the local circumstances.

The ways in which the social work profession has responded to the evidence-based practice movement, the pressures to gather and produce evidence and the need for an accepted knowledge base for practice is the focus of the remaining chapters in this book. The 'gold standard', systematic review process assumes that there is an instrumental relationship between research and practice in terms of 'what works' or 'what works best' rather than an informed interpretation and judgements about appropriate practice responses in light of the range of evidence (Hammersley 2001). As we shall see in Chapter 6, the implementation of evidence-based practice in social work is not a simple instrumental process, but is a political, cultural, bureaucratic and value-driven process. Different international contexts, theoretical perspectives and actor networks are impacting upon the ways in which evidence-based practice is being 'implemented' in social work. That is, the ways in which concepts, information and ways of understanding the world are shaping social work practice and social work research.

Note

1 Behaviourist-decisionism is defined as a methodology that endorses the purely formal structure of decision without regard for the specificity of its content. According to decisionism, it is not the content of the decision, but rather the fact that it is a decision made by an expert authority, or by using a correct method, which determines its validity.

3 Framing social work knowledge

The previous chapters have introduced evidence-based practice (EBP) in the wider context beyond social work, where it is influential in a range of disciplines and in the realms of public policy and service provision. This chapter narrows the focus to what evidence-based practice has come to mean for social work and the process of knowledge formation within the profession. As we suggested in Chapter 1, a broad definition of evidence-based social work entails the mobilization of a specialist research infrastructure to inform particular interventions, support best practice governance and demonstrate positive outcomes for service users. We noted that evidence-based practice *becomes* evidence-based social work at the point when it materializes in a more or less fixed set of locations within social work and is performed and durable. We place an emphasis on the transportability of evidence-based practice *into* social work, based on a series of implementation moves. In this sense, evidence-based practice becomes 'evidence-based social work' through a process of translation.

As the origins of evidence-based practice lie with the medical profession, the early use of evidence-based social work is located with those social work interventions that resemble medical interventions, i.e., standardized treatments implemented in order to achieve defined, desirable outcomes. While this approach to evidence-based practice retains a strong position in social work, the concept of evidence-based social work has evolved beyond this original – some would say purist – perspective.

Knowledge formation is never a uniform, stable or monolithic activity and inevitably it will throw up highly charged, contradictory and contestable debate. Such is the case with the views on the nature of evidence discussed in the previous chapter, where we examined the notion of evidence, including the 'gold standard' paradigm for evidence-based practice and the strengths and limitations of other types of evidence. This chapter goes on to examine the competing methodological claims and theoretical positions that impact upon the formulation of evidence-based social work. Recent developments in the ways in which the social work knowledge base is framed are discussed with regard to the challenges that an evidence-based perspective introduces into social work. Evidence-based social work is presented in the context of the theoretical and ethical traditions that guide and influence the profession of social work.

The evolution of evidence-based social work has been informed by debates about the utility and quality of evidence for social work decision-making. The purist approach to evidence, entailing systematic reviews of randomized controlled trials (RCTs), has not yet met the needs of social workers dealing with complex and varied practices, in different settings and with unique presenting issues (Hall 2008). The social work profession has been examining how evidence-based practice, with the vast resource base it requires to produce 'gold standard' evidence and the questionable usefulness of this evidence to much practice, can be shaped in a meaningful way for the profession (Rubin and Parrish 2007a). Social work practitioners are being required by employers and policy-makers to provide evidence for their practice and to engage in debates about evidence-based practice, but are struggling to understand what evidence-based practice actually means for social work (Murphy and McDonald 2004). For some, this shift from the scientific position on evidence-based social work is seen as a retreat from the ethical obligations of social work and an opportunity to rest in an uncritical way on the established authority of the profession (Gambrill 1999, 2004). In this chapter, we show that rather than being a backward step, the different approaches to evidence-based social work enhance the position of social work in gathering evidence in an ethical and critically reflective way.

In drawing on Plath's (in Gray and Webb 2008a) new framework for identifying the different perspectives on evidence-based practice (see Table 3.1), we examine the theoretical and practice traditions that have influenced evidence-based social work: positivist, pragmatic, political and postmodern. We identify the type of evidence sought, the processes employed, and the relationship between research and practice from each perspective.

Consideration is given in this chapter to the strengths and weaknesses associated with each perspective and the circumstances under which it is most useful for social work to adopt a particular theoretical or practice perspective. The social work profession has a strong values and ethics base which has influenced academic debates about evidence-based social work and the formation of knowledge within the profession. Claims and debates about ethical responsibility associated with each of the four perspectives on evidence-based social work are considered in this chapter. Critical thinking, professional judgement and professional authority are also features of social work practice that have had a role to play in debates about evidence-based social work and are considered in this chapter in regard to each of the four theoretical perspectives in Table 3.1.

The intention in the chapter is to demonstrate that no particular theoretical approach to evidence-based social work is necessarily 'better', but rather that different theoretical approaches may suit different contexts or goals in practice. Critical analysis and ethical responsibility remain fundamental to all approaches and there is not one approach that has a greater claim on these professional principles than any other. The critical thinking and interactive skills of practitioners in making judgements are vital elements in the process of adopting different, evidence-based social work approaches.

Table 3.1 Four theoretical influences on evidence-based practice

Positivist	Pragmatic	Political	Postmodern
Type of evidence sought			
Strong evidence Definitive answers about effectiveness	Useful evidence Relevant information to assist practice decision-making	Influential evidence Information that can be used strategically to obtain resources, further causes, uphold professional ethics and promote practice principles	Evidence as discourse Information that can be used to enhance particular meanings and interpretations of practice and its impact
Processes to generate evidence			
Randomized controlled trials (RCTs) Systematic reviews and meta-analyses	Theoretical and practical synthesis of research findings, incorporating a range of methods Critical reflection on the limitations and applicability of research findings to practice	Strategically chosen and negotiated evidence in contested domains Advocacy, lobbying	Discourse to establish common meaning and interpretation of experiences in the profession, organizations and other social groupings
Relationship between research and practice			
Research directs practice	Symbiotic relationship between research and practice	Research is a tool to achieve professional practice goals, including those based on ethical and value stances	Research and practice both contribute to enhancing the meaning and status of social work

Adapted from Plath (in Gray and Webb 2008a: 180).

Positivist evidence-based social work

We saw in Chapter 1 that a positivist approach to the social sciences developed from the scientific paradigm of the physical sciences. The social world, from a positivist perspective, is real and tangible in the same way that the physical world is. As such, understanding and explanation of social phenomena are gained through systematic observation and measurement. For social work, this means that the effectiveness of interventions is assessed in terms of measurable outcomes. A positivist position on evidence-based social work may be regarded as the pure and original form of evidence-based practice, as it is aligned with the treatment terminology of medicine where evidence-based practice originated. The positivist approach is aligned with the 'gold standard' approach to evidence-based practice, discussed in Chapter 2. This traditional approach entails a hierarchy of evidence, established in terms of the strength of the research methodology to determine relationships between phenomena and causal links between intervention and outcomes.

Evidence-based social work, which is grounded in this positivist perspective, entails the evaluation of standardized interventions using 'gold standard' experimental research methods. A body of research evidence on the effectiveness of interventions is gathered over time and across different contexts. This evidence is made available to practitioners through systematic reviews of effectiveness research. Practitioners and clients are then in a position to make informed choices between interventions in terms of demonstrated effectiveness. A positivist influence is evident within the academic literature on evidence-based social work, in the writing of, among others, Gambrill (1999, 2004, 2006b), Howard *et al.* (2003), Macdonald (2001), McNeece and Thyer (2004), Roberts and Yeager (2006), Sheldon (2001), Thyer (2002), and Thyer and Kazi (2004).

The positivist approach strives for definitive answers about the effectiveness of interventions based on the strongest scientific evidence. By 'strongest' is meant that evidence which is robust, reliable, rigorous and valid. The purpose of this evidence is to guide decisions about the best interventions for clients and where to direct scarce resources for social service provision. Scientific research findings are regarded as information upon which practice decisions should be based and a source of legitimacy and ethical standing for the profession (Thyer and Kazi 2004).

When is a positivist approach appropriate?

The strength of the positivist perspective lies with the robustness of the evidence that can be produced by well-designed experimental studies. It is an enticing prospect for a profession that struggles daily with the complexities and inconsistencies of human, social, political and organizational behaviour to be able to say with definitive authority that one intervention works better than another. While evidence-based social work has moved on from this simplistic view, an accessible body of cumulative evidence resulting from well-designed research, incorporating wide cross-sections of clients from a variety of contexts, would certainly strengthen the profession and considerably clarify decision-making about where to direct energy and money.

In Chapter 2 we argued, however, that not all social work interventions lend themselves to RCT experiments or even to single-system and quasi-experimental designs. This is certainly true for community- and organization-focused interventions, as well as for many client interventions where varying needs and interpersonal dynamics often make it inappropriate to provide the standardized type of interventions required for experimental study. Evidence based on experimental design should not, however, be discarded because of this lack of universal application. RCTs and other experimental designs may be complex and difficult to orchestrate in evaluating social work interventions, but the answers that such studies can produce could offer a degree of confidence in social work and social policy decisions that cannot be provided otherwise. In situations where there are clearly defined interventions, access to large samples (or for single-case designs, multiple testing opportunities), agreement on what constitutes a successful outcome and the potential to identify and control intervening variables, there is an imperative for social work to engage in such research. While much social work practice is reliant on context and interpersonal relationships, this is insufficient reason to ignore the potential for experimental research. Social work practice benefits from the investigation of practice that yields strong evidence for effectiveness, as this evidence can be applied successfully for the benefit of clients and the profession (Macdonald 2001; Roberts and Yeager 2006). The challenge for social work is to identify the interventions that are suitable for experimental evaluation and to consider the applicability of RCT evaluations for a range of intervention types. For example, experimental designs have been used successfully to evaluate the outcomes of distinct labour market and social welfare policy interventions for experimental and control populations (Burtless 2002; Gueron 2002, 2007).

Limitations and prospects for a positivist approach to evidence-based social work

The positivist approach to evidence-based social work has, however, come under criticism for a number of reasons. First, experimental designs have been seen to reduce the complex human experiences encountered by social workers to quantifiable variables that are of limited relevance to real practice experience (Epstein 1996; Shaw 1999; Witkin 1991, 1996). Experimental designs can produce reliable information about unrealistically defined constructs and limited contexts that may not be more widely applicable in social work practice. That is, while the internal validity of the experiment under controlled conditions may be strong, the external validity needed to apply the findings to other contexts can be weak. Ian Shaw (1999) states that while RCTs lead to a greater certainty of results, there needs to be a trade-off between certainty of outcomes and the importance and relevance of the research. It is better for the quality of social work practice, he argues, to have less dependable answers about a broader range of questions. As proponents of experimental design in education, Thomas Cook and Monique Payne (2002: 153) also concede that:

> … experiments were not developed to answer questions about complex causal interdependencies. Their purpose is more narrow and practical – to identify whether one or more possible causal agents actually cause change in a given outcome.

and that:

> … proponents of random assignment need to acknowledge that the method they prefer depends on a theory of causation that is less comprehensive than the more multivariate and explanatory theory that most social scientists espouse.
>
> (*ibid.*: 154)

The positivist approach may also be criticized because of the limited applicability of experimental designs to the evaluation of much social work intervention. Social work interventions are generally not specifically defined and standardized interventions, but are adapted and combined to respond to presenting issues. In social work practice, the 'same' intervention never gets implemented identically and never has the same impact, because of differences in the context, setting, process and stakeholders. This lack of standardization does not suit the controlled requirements of experimental designs. The implication of this situation may be that certain interventions are not given attention by evidence-seekers, not because the interventions are ineffective but rather because the nature of the intervention does not lend itself to the experimental designs that will generate acceptable evidence. Collaborative, developmental interventions with clients and communities that are responsive to emerging needs and issues, for example, are unlikely to be examined by experimental studies. The positivist approach to evidence-based social work may bring into question 'bottom-up' community development, participatory or empowerment practices where discrete interventions and outcomes are hard to define, and promote interventions that are limited and standardized, even when local conditions require a diversity of responses (Hausman 2002). A review of the volume edited by Albert Roberts and Kenneth Yeager (2006) indicates that standardized, psychological, therapeutic interventions, such as cognitive behaviour therapy (CBT), attract most attention in scientific evidence-based practice reviews, which brings into question whether it is the profession of social work or psychology for which evidence is being gathered.

Another limitation of the positivist approach is that experimental designs to evaluate outcomes require a defined and agreed understanding of an effective outcome and how this is measured. What is deemed to be an 'effective' outcome of a social worker's intervention, however, is often difficult to define and measure. While there may be a common core of agreement about desired outcomes – e.g., to obtain employment – intervention outcomes tend to be multi-faceted in response to multiple presenting needs, e.g., to improve mental health and access suitable child care in order to obtain and maintain employment. The definition of effectiveness can also vary with the standpoint of the person evaluating the practice and the particular context. The goals against which effectiveness is judged are essentially linked to the values guiding the assessment of the presenting issues. Juliet Cheetham (1992) draws a useful distinction between the service provider perspective – 'quality of care' – and the client experience – 'quality of life'. A successful outcome may look quite different from these two perspectives. For much social work practice, there are multiple desirable outcomes possible. Experimental designs can create an ethical conflict for social work by focusing attention on assessing particular outcomes, while other issues for the client are ignored (Epstein 1996).

The feasibility of using a positivist approach in evidence-based social work is questionable because of the substantial economic and training resources required to support this type of evidence base for social work. The inadequacy of research evidence to inform social work practice continues to be identified in the literature (Cheetham 1992, 1997; Gibbs and Gambrill 2002; Gilgun 2005; Macdonald and Sheldon 1992; Mullen, Bellamy *et al.* 2005; Scott 2002; Shaw 2003; Sheldon 1986).

Given the vast array of social work contexts, client groups and interventions, the task of conducting comprehensive and high-quality research studies and systematic reviews to support social work practice is overwhelming. While the availability of research evidence is increasing, most social work practice decisions must still be based upon non-empirical knowledge (Reid 2001). The results of meta-analyses of research and systematic reviews of literature on social work-related issues are often found to be inconclusive (Zlotnik *et al.* 2005). The availability of research findings that are widely useful and applicable to social workers internationally is an optimistic expectation that we are currently a long way from achieving. Dissemination of research findings and systematic reviews through internet-based organizations – such as the Cochrane Collaboration, Campbell Collaboration, and Social Care Institute for Excellence (SCIE) – make access to findings much easier than it was in the past for social workers. But, as social, economic, political and organizational contexts change, the nature of presenting issues, practice responses and intervention goals also shift for social work. The process of reviewing, compiling and updating findings for internet access by social workers thus becomes a continuous and highly resource-intensive one (Warburton and Black 2002).

A related challenge is to facilitate the use of existing research findings by social workers to inform their practice. Social workers tend to make very little use of research findings and, when they do draw on research, there is a tendency to alter the reported intervention to fit their own practice context (Reid 2001). The wider availability of research evidence may not prompt social workers to practise differently, as practice decision-making incorporates much more complex processes than having research evidence at hand (Webb 2001, 2002). Time, inclination and research ability are also factors contributing to social workers' reluctance to use research.

Macdonald (2001: 25) states that the potential for evidence-based social work relies upon five conditions:

1 investment in good quality research;
2 access to summaries of research, good quality systematic reviews and meta-analyses;
3 ability of practitioners to make use of evidence in practice;
4 ability to employ the skills and services indicated by the evidence;
5 ability to monitor, review and change practice.

The evidence-based practice movement in social work still has a long way to go before these conditions are sufficiently met. Considerable resources, organizational support, training and encouragement are required before a useful body of experimental research could be made available as social work evidence.

Positivism and ethical responsibility

Social work as a profession is well grounded in ethical principles and, consequently, ethical concerns have shaped debates around experimental designs and the adoption of a positivist approach to gathering evidence for social work. Arguments for evidence-based social work from a positivist perspective have included the ethical responsibility of social workers to have strong and reliable evidence about the most effective and beneficial services for clients. Such evidence is required, it is argued, in order to justify intervening in people's lives and using public monies to do so (Ainsworth and Hansen 2005; Cheetham 1992; Macdonald 2001; Sheldon 1986; Thyer and Kazi 2004). As a counter-argument to this ethical stance, the identification and promotion of 'best practices' supported by an evidence base could lead to a reduction in the range of services available to clients and hence act as a threat to client self-determination (Hausman 2002). Eileen Gambrill (2004: 218), however, claims that, with rigorous appraisals of practice-related research findings, the potential for clients to make informed choices will be increased:

> Many clients and consumers will learn to ask questions such as 'What are my alternatives?' 'How do their outcomes compare with services you recommend?' 'How accurate is this test?' 'What is the rate of false positives?' 'Are there any harmful effects of what you recommend?

Ethical responsibility may also be raised in regard to the conduct of experimental studies needed in order to gather evidence (Epstein 1996). One of the features of an experimental study is the comparison of an experimental group that receives a particular intervention with a control group that does not. A consequence of this design is that one group will miss out on a potentially helpful intervention. This denial of service to a group in need poses an ethical concern. The reality of social service provision is, however, that many people are denied services due to the limits on resources available. Decisions are made about which people should and should not receive services on the basis of sometimes subjective definitions of need. It has been argued, by proponents of experimental designs, that random assignment to control and experimental groups is, therefore, no less detrimental than existing arrangements (Cook and Payne 2002). Concern about denial of services is overcome if the service being evaluated is specially funded for the purpose of the evaluation (Gueron 2002). In such cases, the experimental group is in receipt of enriched services that would not otherwise be available. The control group remains entitled to the full range of services that are generally available in the community. Another approach to dealing with ethical concerns with experiments is the use of a cross-over design, which involves the control group being offered treatment after the experimental phase is complete (Cook and Payne 2002). This design may be used in situations where a delay in treatment is not of great concern.

Experimental designs may also be challenged because of the untested and potentially harmful interventions that people are exposed to and the high costs of quality experimental studies when money is needed for service provision to clients. Proponents of experimental designs argue that the alternative is for social workers to continue to use finite resources and to expose clients to untested and potentially detrimental practices in their daily work. Despite the ethical tensions associated with experimental designs, it is these fundamental ethical concerns that drive the desire for strong evidence through experimental social work studies (Macdonald and Sheldon 1992; Sheldon 1986; Thyer and Kazi 2004).

Critical thinking, professional judgement and professional authority within a positivist perspective

One of the strengths of an evidence-based practice approach is that it requires a critical approach to practice. Evidence-based practice involves the 'questioning of unfounded beliefs, rigorous scrutiny of methodology and critical appraisal of proposed treatments' (Bilsker and Goldner 2000: 664). Practitioners are compelled to adopt a critical and questioning approach to accepted practices and to examine the relative effectiveness of these practices in the context of other possible interventions. More importantly, they are required to critically appraise the quality of research. On the basis of the rigour that is applied in experimental designs and systematic reviews, proponents of a positivist approach to evidence-based social work have laid claim to the practice of critical thinking about evidence or critical appraisal of evidence. The location of critical thinking solely within the realm of science is certainly open to dispute. It was noted in Chapter 1 that Gambrill (1999) proposes that the alternative to an evidence-based approach is an authority-based approach that relies on professional status and untested assumptions. Similarly, Thyer and Kazi (2004: 4) suggest that the alternative to a scientific approach to evidence is 'rhetoric, authority, theory, power or tradition to support artificially one's personal views'. The positivist assumption in such statements is that evidence from scientific research is 'real' and personal views are 'artificial'. This extends to an assumption that critical appraisal can relate only to the evaluation of research, but not to that of personal and professional views. It is assumptions such as these that have been the source of much concern and debate in the social work profession. In contrast to the views of Gambrill and Thyer and Kazi, it is apparent that just as personal views can be held uncritically, so too can research findings be adopted uncritically or to gain professional legitimacy. Effective social work practice relies upon critical thinking and reflection about both personal views and research findings, and also about the range of theoretical, political, interpersonal and ethical dimensions that contribute to professional judgements.

Evidence-based practice is concerned with critically reviewing accepted practices and incorporating new knowledge. There is, however, resistance – among some who hold on to the scientific paradigm – to reconsidering this model for evidence-based practice in social work. Gambrill (2004: 215) expresses concern that 'practices are being labelled as "evidence-based" which have few if any of the hallmarks of the philosophy and technology of EBP as described by its originators'. It was pointed out in Chapter 1 that Gambrill's own perspective suffers from the very same complaint she makes about other contributions to the field of evidence-based social work. However, we concur that, in line with evidence-based practice principles, we should embrace this opportunity for critique, critically question the accepted authority of the scientific paradigm and carefully assess other approaches to evidence-based social work.

Social work has a strong and well-developed tradition of critical reflection on personal, interpersonal and political factors. Self-reflection and awareness of personal values and biases are fundamental to social work training. The radical, feminist, structural and critical theory traditions in social work have questioned professional status and authority (see Gray and Webb 2008a). To claim that the alternative to a scientific approach to social work practice is to rely uncritically on personal views and professional authority is unreasonable in light of these traditions in social work. It is these theoretical and practice traditions in social work that have influenced the way in which evidence-based practice has been shaped and enhanced (not eroded, as those who do not acknowledge the limitations of positivism may claim). Pragmatic, political and postmodern influences on evidence-based social work are discussed in the subsequent sections.

Pragmatic evidence-based social work

A pragmatic approach to evidence-based social work acknowledges the limited application of experimental research in social work. It proposes that findings from experimental research should be incorporated with a range of other information, knowledge and theoretical understandings in making professional judgements about practice interventions. A pragmatic approach is mindful of the realities and constraints of professional social work practice. The emphasis is upon identifying useful evidence that realistically can be gathered and applied by social workers needing to make informed judgements in particular practice contexts. It is the relevance and applicability of the research that is regarded as being of greater importance than the particular methodological approach used. A pragmatic approach to evidence-based practice is evident in writing by Shaw (1999, 2003), Newman and McNeish (2005), Plath (2006), and in the edited volume by Smith (2004).

A pragmatic approach does not mean that any available information is accepted uncritically. Information that is gathered should be critically evaluated in terms of strengths, limitations and applicability to the practice setting. It is recognized that the findings of RCTs are context dependent and, while contributing potentially useful information about that controlled context, are not necessarily the most relevant information for particular presenting issues in another context. From a pragmatic viewpoint, research should be accessible and integrated with practice. Research is designed in line with what is realistic, achievable and relevant to practice. As such, small onsite studies are valued for their local relevance and insights. Practitioners require skills in undertaking practice-based research, synthesizing and critically evaluating research and analyzing a range of practice and contextual factors in order to make informed judgements, rather than definitive claims about their own practice. Research-based practice and practice-based research models reflect a pragmatic approach to the integration of research with the requirements of daily practice in social work.

A pragmatic approach aims to address the complex and multi-dimensional nature of social work practice by moving beyond narrow questions associated with experimental design, such as: is X effective? or does X work better than Y? Research evidence that is useful for social work deals with the more detailed questions, such as: what aspects worked well? what aspects didn't work well? why? how did people experience the intervention? in what ways did these experiences differ? and what were the factors impacting upon these experiences? Evidence for social work practice entails more than studying the outcomes and effectiveness of interventions, but should also examine the processes involved in these interventions (Rubin and Parrish 2007a). A combination of qualitative and quantitative methods and enquiry from a variety of perspectives is, therefore, promoted in order to investigate the complexities of social work practice.

While clear differences exist between the positivist and pragmatic approaches in terms of notions of 'best evidence', there remains an area of agreement between the two approaches to evidence-based social work. The common ground is a general agreement in the social work literature that appropriate methods must be chosen for the social work research questions being asked and that a range of different research methods, both qualitative and quantitative, can contribute to the advancement of social work knowledge. While promoting the explanatory role of controlled experiments, Reid (2001), for example, also states that qualitative research is needed in order to develop and test theories and to better understand complex phenomena. There is an emphasis in social work research literature on the need for mixed-method approaches (Cheetham 1992, 1997; Gibbs 2001; Reid 2001; Shaw 1999, 2003; Sheldon 1986). The difference is that, from a positivist perspective, experimental evidence is regarded as the best evidence that should be produced if at all possible, whereas from a pragmatic perspective, all research evidence needs to be weighed alongside other sources of information and insights in order for practitioners to make informed judgements about interventions. It is accepted by the pragmatist that experimental designs and systematic reviews may determine answers to some social work questions. Generally, however, social workers are faced with questions where there are no definitive answers. The pragmatist argues that social workers need a varied range of information in order to critically examine practice and to support and justify decision-making.

When is a pragmatic approach appropriate?

One of the strengths of a pragmatic approach is that social workers are able to build a balanced picture of the practice issue of concern by drawing on process and outcome data, practice wisdom of colleagues, personal experience, and client feedback. Social workers can examine multiple questions and a range of perspectives on the effectiveness of practice. Research findings are integrated with existing social work knowledge in critically evaluating future directions for practice. A further strength of the pragmatic approach is that it is concerned with current presenting practice issues in real organizational contexts. It promotes practical strategies for accessing information to inform the practice issue and is realistic about the limitations on evidence for practice. As such, it is suited to the demands of daily practice in organizational settings where issues need to be resolved in efficient and meaningful ways. The pragmatist trades off definitive answers for the ability to make informed judgements about immediate, complex practice issues in particular contexts. This is evidence-based social work for the busy practitioner, rather than for the research scholar.

Limitations and prospects for a pragmatic approach to evidence-based social work

The priority given by the pragmatist to gathering evidence in response to current practice issues may be criticized for being short-sighted. In order to build a body of evidence from which social workers can draw, a longer-term view is needed that entails building a bank of evidence about a wide range of social work questions and issues. While the pragmatist places fewer limitations than the positivist on what is deemed to be suitable evidence, concerns about the lack of high-quality social work research upon which practitioners can draw is also a major concern if a pragmatic approach to evidence-based social work were to succeed. When a pragmatic approach is used to deal with a presenting practice issue and no relevant, quality research findings are available, social workers may only have personal experiences and client feedback to draw upon. While this is still useful evidence from a pragmatic perspective, it is limited on its own and falls short of the balanced appraisal of a range of evidence that is the goal of a pragmatic approach. The realities of frontline practice can be that practitioners, under pressure to produce evidence, will grasp any available information, despite its shortfalls and limitations, and present this as the evidence. In Chapter 1 we suggested that this lends itself more accurately to a form of information-based rather than evidence-based practice in social work. It is this type of 'anything goes' approach, given an 'evidence-based' label by practitioners and policy-makers under pressure, that has been strongly criticized by the positivists who maintain high standards on research design (Gambrill 2004).

Another concern with the pragmatic approach is that the requirement for evidence to be assessed in terms of relevance and applicability to a particular practice context offers limited guidance to practitioners. Creativity and lateral thinking come into play, along with critical thinking in examining relevance and applicability of research findings. There is some latitude and room for interpretation in this process, allowing for evidence to be biased toward particular preferences. While the goal of the pragmatist is the appraisal of available evidence from a range of sources, the actual process may be a biased and haphazard one. The social worker who is not skilled in critiquing research may be swayed by reported research findings without appraising these critically. The pragmatic approach could also be used as a rationale for ignoring empirical research altogether and to draw only on the experiences of direct practice.

For pragmatic evidence-based social work to achieve its objectives, there is a need to address the barriers to social workers accessing and applying research findings. When social workers are aware of the ways in which research evidence can be useful for practice, they are more likely to access this information. The availability of quality research, the level of motivation to use research evidence and skill base of social workers will need to be enhanced in order to avoid the risk that pragmatic evidence-based social work will become an excuse to ignore research altogether.

Ethical responsibility and pragmatism

While the pragmatic approach to evidence-based social work may not encounter the same type of ethical concerns levelled against experimental designs, ethical concerns about the invasive nature of much research remain. Ethical responsibility may be addressed by ensuring informed consent of participants, promoting participatory research and maintaining the overriding principle that all of the research that is conducted must be useful in informing and guiding better quality practice in the future. The high cost of experimental studies is reduced by promoting a range of research designs, including small, practice-based research projects. If useful information for improving practice can be gathered through less costly and less invasive means, then, ethically, it is these that should be chosen.

Critical thinking, professional judgement and professional authority within a pragmatist perspective

In order for pragmatic evidence-based social work to maintain integrity and avoid declining into an 'any evidence will do' approach, social workers need to be rigorous, critical thinkers at various stages in the process. In gathering evidence, social workers should be thorough in seeking out and compiling information from all available sources. This entails lateral thinking and meticulous searching skills as information relevant to a practice decision is gathered from a diverse range of sources. Social workers require skills in the critical appraisal of research studies, including a range of research designs. Equally important are the critical appraisal skills needed to assess the applicability of findings to a particular practice context and to translate these into improved practice. Training and organizational support will increase the capacity of social workers to engage successfully in these processes. Social workers are required to analyze the interpersonal, social, cultural, political, economic and organizational factors in a particular practice context and to assess the ways in which these may impact upon the nature of interventions and the outcomes for the client. Findings from research studies then become one component in a more complex process of critical reflection and professional judgement about appropriate practice interventions. Importantly, the pragmatist accepts that many social work practice questions will not be answered fully and that judgements without definitive evidence will remain the reality of much social work practice that deals with unique, dynamic and complex scenarios. Practice decisions are made on the balance of evidence and in light of ethical and theoretical principles, professional skills, interpersonal dynamics and contextual analysis.

Political evidence-based social work

A political approach to evidence-based social work is grounded in the social work tradition of responding to powerlessness and marginalization as the focus of practice. As Michael Sheppard (2006) conveys, concern for the exclusion and powerlessness of individuals and groups in society has been a defining feature of social work. The political approach is influenced by the group of radical, feminist and structural theories that have had a longstanding impact on the knowledge base of social work (Bailey and Brake 1975; Corrigan and Leonard 1978; Fook 1993; Gray and Webb 2008b; Mullaly 2007). Fundamental to the political approach to evidence-based social work is recognition that there are differences in the power and influence of groups in society and that the role of social work is to negotiate oppressive systems with the goal of empowering marginalized groups. The political perspective offers both a critique and a way forward in evidence-based social work. Some authors who have integrated a political analysis in writings about evidence-based practice are Dore (2006), Morse (2006), Pawson (2006) and Plath (2006).

From a political perspective, the processes involved in gathering and presenting evidence for particular interventions are not accepted as the rigorous, technical processes that they can be made out to be. Evidence-gathering and knowledge-formation processes are considered in the wider political context and examined in terms of how they reflect the power differences and dynamics that are the features of social life. The role of political evidence-based practice is first to expose such biases and second, to promote the voices of marginalized and socially excluded people as sources of evidence.

Some of the decisions that may exclude certain marginalized perspectives, but nonetheless impact on the body of evidence produced for social work, include decisions about how much funding there is for social work research, the types of research that are funded, the organizations that are funded to do research, the interventions that are evaluated, the research methods employed, how research findings are disseminated, the 'social issues' that are identified as worthy of research, the ways in which 'effectiveness' is defined, and the relative value that each different type of research evidence is given. A political view of evidence-based social work recognizes that gathering and presenting evidence is one of the arenas of social work practice that must be handled strategically in order to ensure that the social work goals of empowerment and social inclusion remain fundamental. Evidence can be gathered to advance the causes of professionals, organizations and research institutes or used strategically to provide opportunities for the voices of less powerful groups, including service users, to have some influence in social work practice and social policy decision-making.

The political context of social work shapes practices, priorities and decision-making. From a political perspective, evidence that is likely to be influential in a given context is sought from a variety of sources. The evidence is used strategically to raise awareness of issues for disadvantaged and marginalized groups and to influence the distribution of resources. Evidence is gathered as one of the tools that may be used in negotiating power relationships through advocacy and lobbying in contested domains.

When is a political approach appropriate?

One of the strengths of the political approach is that it addresses the fact that research alone will not achieve change. If change in service provision were to occur, the relevance and implications of research would need to be used to persuade decision-makers and funding bodies. The political approach provides a clear focus and purpose for that change, which is closely aligned with the social justice goals of social work. It also requires that social workers consider the power dynamics and processes involved in convincing decision-makers, at organizational and policy levels, that this evidence is 'real' and needs to be taken seriously.

By examining the wider political and economic context of research funding and research priorities, the political perspective directs attention to bias in resource distribution and the types of evidence that become privileged through such processes (e.g., particular methods, research populations and interventions evaluated). One of the concerns about evidence-based practice, expressed within the social work profession, has been that the language of outcomes and effectiveness reflects managerial values of optimizing outputs and ensuring value for money, which does not always fit with social work values (Gibbs 2001; Webb 2001). A particular service or policy direction may be given legitimacy as 'evidence-based' if available research were to suggest that good outcomes would result. Likewise, a service may be withdrawn if no such evidence is available or the only available measure of effectiveness is in terms of cost. In light of the paucity of available research, this risk gives cause for concern. The broader level of analysis offered by a political perspective on evidence-based practice gives social workers a framework for analysis and debate on these issues.

A political approach directs attention toward the interventions and population groups that are being overlooked in the allocation of research monies. It promotes research and information-gathering techniques, such as feminist and action research models, that are participatory and emancipatory in nature. The political approach seeks out evidence for innovation, newly emerging issues and marginalized perspectives.

Debate about the definition of the 'effectiveness' of social work interventions is a practice issue that might also benefit from a political perspective. Within government departments and social service organizations, decisions about service funding are influenced by perceptions of the effectiveness of services. Regardless of how rigorous and definitive the research evidence for outcomes of an intervention might be, this would have little impact on decision-makers if there were no common agreement on what constituted an effective outcome. Despite the efforts of social workers and researchers to establish effectiveness, research findings could be disregarded. The reality of service funding trends is that, even with an increased interest in research by policy-makers, policy and practice changes tend to be incremental and take little account of research findings (Cheetham 1992,

1997; Harries *et al.* 1999). Social workers need to engage in awareness-raising, lobbying and coalition-building activities to influence understanding of how an effective outcome would look from the client or consumer perspective. The social worker might need to campaign over a period of time to challenge narrow views of effectiveness defined exclusively in terms of cost efficiency. With empowerment and social inclusion as underlying principles for practice, the social worker has a responsibility to ensure that client experiences are central in understanding practice effectiveness and in the evidence that is presented. Gibbs (2001) argues that the trend toward short-term, outcome-based, 'good-enough' information for agencies can lead to important feedback from service users being ignored. In such an environment, there is a risk that the cost-efficiency goals of management would prevail in definitions of effectiveness. A political approach to challenging and presenting evidence is a role for social work and, as Cheetham (1992) signals, when effectiveness is argued convincingly, policy-makers might not necessarily choose the cheapest option.

Limitations and prospects for a political approach to evidence-based social work

A feature of the political approach is in the biased way in which social workers may identify the causes that they pursue and the evidence they consequently promote. Personal and social biases can influence which groups are perceived by the social workers as worthy of their strategic lobbying and advocacy activities. While this could be perceived as a weakness in the approach, it can also be viewed as the nature of participation in the social world. As lobby groups and consumer groups advocate for a range of disadvantaged groups that tussle for recognition in society, the realm of marginalization is also a contested political domain. Deciding which group's interests to promote might present ethical dilemmas, not to mention the conflicts of interest between groups. If research evidence were used as a strategic political tool, the substance and quality of the research might become less important than its impact and influence in political decision-making. The political approach would need to be combined with an open-minded ability to locate, critique and synthesize research evidence, along with critical self-reflection, if it were to be more than game-playing using the language of evidence as a hollow political tool.

The challenge is to integrate a political approach with strong research analysis skills. For example, Judith Gueron (2002) argues that while random assignment offers the greatest certainty of any research method, the experimental design is just the first step. Drawing on her own experiences of successful experimental designs to evaluate policy interventions, she asserts that operational and political skills are required to interpret and promote the findings before any change is likely to occur. Political astuteness – i.e., skills in negotiation, engagement and influence – is required when working with relevant players to implement the changes indicated by the research findings.

Ethical responsibility and the political approach

The political approach to evidence-based social work is well grounded in the fundamental social work value of promoting social justice, part of which is working to empower disadvantaged and marginalized groups. Within this approach, providing opportunities for marginalized voices to be heard is an underlying principle in both the conduct of research and the strategic use of evidence. Clients' rights, participation and self-determination have become issues of debate in relation to research in social work, with experimental approaches and outcomes-based research being associated with a negation of consumer participation in research (Gibbs 2001). What is found in the research to 'work' may not be what clients desire or believe that they need (Hausman 2002). In such situations, should the worker be 'evidence-based' or 'client-centred'? In support of experimental methods, Gambrill (1999), as discussed above, argues that clients must become active participants in decision-making by being presented with intervention alternatives and given the research evidence on effectiveness in order to make their decision. Such clearly defined and evidenced choices are, however, unlikely to occur in practice. Often practitioners are faced with the struggle of finding any support service, rather than having a choice between different services. The political approach seeks to address such inadequacies by promoting the concerns of marginalized groups as evidence for practice.

Critical thinking, professional judgement and professional authority within a political perspective

A political approach to evidence-based social work requires a critical thinking and analytical capacity in appraising the range of factors – economic, social, cultural, political and so on – that impact upon the creation and promotion of evidence for practice. Critical analysis skills are also required in assessing interactional dynamics and determining strategies that might influence decision-makers and draw attention to disadvantaged groups. Social workers need to examine closely the strengths and limitations of research evidence. Regardless of how strong the evidence for a particular intervention might be, social workers are in a position where they must critically reflect on their work in the political, social, organizational and interpersonal contexts, make professional judgements, engage in debate with decision-makers about resource allocation, negotiate appropriate practices and, when necessary, argue convincingly for the effectiveness of the work that is done. This requires skills in formulating and presenting well-supported arguments and the interpersonal and written communication skills to convey a position convincingly (see Gray and McDonald 2006).

Postmodern evidence-based social work

Discussion on the way in which knowledge is framed in the social work profession would not be complete without consideration being given to the influence of the postmodern perspective on social work and, consequently, on evidence-based social work. A postmodern influence manifests in the way that social work recognizes and values interpretation, and the subjective meanings and experiences of individuals, cultural groups and societies. While postmodernism has been conveyed in a range of complex ways, essentially a postmodern approach asserts that the social world is open to interpretation and that meaning is created through the use of language, discourse and symbolism. An outcome of postmodernism is seen in the influential body of literature on critical social work theory (Allan *et al.* 2003; Gray and Webb 2008b; Fawcett, in Gray and Webb 2008a; McBeath and Webb 1991; Pease and Fook 1999).

There does, however, appear to be a basic conflict between postmodernism and evidence-based practice. A postmodern perspective holds that 'intervention', 'success', 'effectiveness' and 'best evidence' are all open to interpretation, and hence it seems contradictory to suggest that research could provide direction for practice. While a postmodern approach is in conflict with a strictly positivist view on evidence-based practice, postmodernism has nonetheless influenced the shaping of a social work approach to evidence-based practice. Writing on evidence-based social work has recognized that the meanings of terms, such as 'intervention', 'effectiveness' and 'evidence', are established through discourse among those engaged with social work. The postmodern influence on evidence-based social work has questioned the positivist view on the social world and argued that all evidence is open to interpretation. The meaning and influence of evidence is negotiated through discourse between relevant players. Such an interpretive approach that recognizes the value of meaning and experience in establishing social work evidence is found in writings on evidence-based social work by Ian Shaw (1999, 2003), David Smith (2004) and Stephen Webb (2002). The postmodern influence is apparent in the expectation that practitioners 'develop a sense of humility, a realisation that our hold on truth is partial, tentative and open to revision' (Bilsker and Goldner 2000: 667).

From a postmodern perspective, evidence is not established through observation and measurement, but rather, evidence is established through discourse. Information is gathered and used to enhance particular meanings and interpretations of practice and to establish a common understanding of its impact. The focus is upon the ways in which discourse is used to frame accepted knowledge and interpret experiences in the profession, organizations and other social groupings. The main research method involves the deconstruction, analysis and interpretation of text, such as interview transcripts, social work records, minutes of meetings, and so on. Using the language of evidence, both research and practice aim to contribute to enhancing the meaning and status of social work.

When is a postmodern approach appropriate?

The benefit of a postmodern perspective for evidence-based social work is that it acknowledges the meanings given to experiences by recipients of social work services. By recognizing that there are many voices in a discourse and ways of understanding, it acknowledges that the clients' views are as valuable as the social workers' and researchers' views. Regardless of the measured outcomes of social work interventions, it is the lived experiences and quality of life of clients that are the real tests of social work effectiveness. This type of information is essentially interpretive in nature, and evidence about the impact of social work can only be gathered using qualitative, interpretive and narrative methods. Such evidence, it is thought, has the potential to provide a much broader and holistic picture of social work's impact. The postmodernist perspective has required that social work incorporate wider definitions of evidence for practice than the originators of evidence-based practice envisaged for the medical context for which it was designed.

A positivist approach to evidence, as discussed above, is suited to standardized social work interventions that have clearly defined and observable desired outcomes measured for effectiveness. For most social work practice, however, outcomes, such as improved 'well-being', increased 'fairness' and enhanced 'social justice', cannot be measured. These concepts are open to a broad range of interpretations, as they are dependent upon values, personal experiences and social context. They are, nonetheless, vital goals, central to clients' interests and to the moral and ethical practice of social work. The nature of the intervention, though centred on client needs, will vary according to the issues and goals that emerge, the skills of the worker, the quality of the relationship between the client and the social worker, and the context of social service provision. In making practice decisions, the social worker is likely to draw on a range of information, values, theories, ideologies, models, procedures, approaches, perspectives and techniques. From a postmodern perspective, a qualitative, interpretive approach to evidence-gathering is often needed, not as second-rate evidence to supplement randomized experiments, but as the only meaningful type of evidence for the experiences associated with social work practice (Fawcett and Featherstone 1998; Fawcett *et al.* 2000).

The postmodern perspective is also useful in analyzing the way in which the language of evidence is used within the social work profession and organizations providing social work services (White, in Gray and Webb 2008a). The language of evidence may be used to shape accepted knowledge and practices and, consequently, to give meaning and status to the profession. The analysis of language and interactions can also be helpful in understanding the positioning of particular, favoured interventions in the practice of social work.

Limitations and prospects for a postmodern approach to evidence-based social work

A criticism that is made of a postmodern approach is that it reflects a relativist view of the world that supports an 'anything goes' approach to evidence, leaving the opportunity for powerful groups to continue to exercise authority (Atherton and Bolland 2003; Gambrill 2006b; Gray and Lovat 2006). Poor research design, small sample sizes and a lack of generalizability of findings in many qualitative research studies have reinforced the view that research from a postmodern perspective serves the purpose of affirming existing professional discourses with little empirical support (Shek *et al.* 2005). As revealed in Chapter 2, poor research design is also common in experimental studies, but apparently not to the detriment of the research method itself. There is a strong and well-established qualitative research methodology discipline that promotes rigorous, reflective and grounded approaches to qualitative research design and data analysis. The onus is upon social work researchers engaged in gathering qualitative evidence to ensure that studies are well designed and rigorously executed in order to carry weight as evidence. The tension between positivist and relativist views of the world has, however, been longstanding in social work and the social sciences more generally. Not surprisingly, this has not been resolved in relation to evidence-based social work.

Ethical responsibility and the postmodern approach

A postmodern perspective on evidence-based social work is supported by the social work ethical principle of respecting diverse individual and cultural experiences. Social work promotes the acceptance of different views, perspectives and experiences and this can be accommodated within a postmodern approach to evidence-based social work. Rather than simply claiming that intervention X works better than intervention Y, a postmodern approach allows for an exploration of the experiences of interventions X and Y and how these may be shaped by different worldviews and their transferability to other cultural contexts. It also provides the scope to examine the experiences of those for whom intervention X does not work better and why this may be. Qualitative and interpretive research methods offer a way to explore such complexities in social work interventions and their impact.

Critical thinking, professional judgement and professional authority within a postmodern perspective

When interpretation and meaning are given centre stage in framing knowledge for the profession, there is a requirement on the social work practitioner constantly to assess and appraise the impact of language, values, interactions and contextual factors in practice. This is in line with the emphasis on the reflective use of self, which is an important part of social work training and practice (D'Cruz *et al.* 2007; Fook 2002; Gould and Taylor 1996; Gray 2007; Ixer 1999; Payne 2002). The evidence-based practice movement has created pressures for social workers in the field to produce scientific evidence for particular practices, when practice experience may suggest that this type of evidence is not conveying the full picture of social work effectiveness. Evidence-based social work can benefit from closer critical reflection on how evidence may be interpreted differently from various perspectives. The interpretive elements of a postmodern perspective are evident in the critical reflective emphasis on reframing, imagination, experiences and feelings, as each unique and complex situation is responded to in practice. Such practice reflection is an important source of evidence for effective practice (Fook 2002; Payne 2002). From a postmodern perspective, it is believed that a critically reflective approach to evidence-based social work would offer a more complex and realistic understanding of evidence through continually analyzing the impact of values, relationships, context, and past experiences and feelings in seeking to understand research findings as they apply to individuals and society.

Where to for evidence-based social work?

Having teased apart theoretical influences shaping evidence-based practice for social work, it is worth considering whether these four approaches as conceived by Plath (2008) are consistent or oppositional, and whether there is potential to integrate them into a holistic understanding of evidence-based practice for the social work profession. In discussing each perspective above in turn, we have identified aspects of social work decision-making for which each is appropriate and useful, but also where the limitations may lie. While certain social work writers on evidence-based practice have been associated here with particular theoretical influences, the truth is that there are probably no purists from any of the four theoretical approaches. Most authors on evidence-based social work recognize that social work, given its nature, requires multiple perspectives and approaches in continuing to build knowledge for practice. The intersection of research evidence with practice context, client preferences and practitioner expertise is well established within social work understanding of evidence-based practice, along with an acceptance of uncertainty about many aspects of interventions (Soydan 2008; see Chapter 4).

Social workers at policy, management and direct practice levels are in the position where they can choose between or integrate the different approaches to evidence-based social work, depending upon the demands of the context. Critical analysis and reflective decision-making, in the face of conflicting ethical and theoretical principles, is not new to social work practice. Social workers manage the contradictions of positivist, pragmatic, political and interpretive approaches as part of daily practice. Social work assessments rely on facts as well as different values and personal interpretations. Decisions about interventions are shaped by empowerment principles as well as by organizational constraints. While in abstract theoretical terms the positivist and interpretive paradigms are distinct, in daily practice social workers draw upon both types of information and more. Likewise, in gathering and applying evidence, social workers can be informed by different theoretical perspectives as they make assessments about best evidence in the presenting scenario. This is far from an 'anything goes' approach, as it requires a critically reflective stance to weighing the strengths and limitations of each approach, as herein suggested, before making a judgement. This is a process of reflective and informed judgement that acknowledges the reality that social workers will not achieve definitive answers to many practice questions. The centrality of human relationships and the diverse and complex contexts in social work practice mean that the integration of scientific, practical, political and interpretive evidence will generally require creativity and improvization on the part of the practitioner (Graybeal 2007).

A critical realist perspective for evidence-based social work

Incorporation of the four theoretical perspectives outlined in this chapter is apparent in some literature on evidence-based practice. For example, the critical realist perspective of Ray Pawson (2006), Sue Clegg (2005) and Nick Tilley (Pawson and Tilley 1997) has made an original contribution to discussion and debate on evidence-based practice and is important for social work to consider. This perspective draws on Roy Bhaskar's (1975) work on scientific realism and, in relation to evidence-based practice, brings together positive features from each of the four perspectives described above. The proponents of critical realism contend that interpretation provides greater explanatory power *vis-à-vis* current research practices and that by using two realist concepts – 'generative mechanism' and 'context' – a number of misinterpretations of RCTs from within the dominant empiricist paradigm can be rectified. Generative mechanisms in realist analysis are described by Pawson (2006: 23) as 'engines of explanation' that allow us to make 'rough sense' of the world, based on what we have learnt about the 'demi-regularities' that exist. Rather than aiming for definitive answers, the critical realist acknowledges that there will be inconsistencies and gaps in knowledge and that generative mechanisms offer a rough guide that enables one to make sense of relationships in the social world. As new information is gathered, these generative mechanisms are refined and adapted. Research synthesis is guided by existing generative mechanisms, together with critical appraisal skills and this process works, in turn, to refine the generative mechanisms.

Instead of searching for generalizable lessons or universal truths, a critical realist approach recognizes and directly addresses the fact that the 'same' intervention never gets implemented identically and never has the same impact, because of differences in the context, setting, process, stakeholders and outcomes. Instead, the aim of realist methodology is explanatory: it asks 'What works for whom, in what circumstances, in what respects, and how?' Pawson (2006) proposes that research should be synthesized in a way that is both theory driven and theory building. Research is reviewed in order to prompt the reconsideration of theoretical understandings that inform service provision and to better understand the complex nature of the context of service provision. Applicability and usefulness are basic principles in the review of research findings, where there is a focus on informing practice decisions. As Pawson *et al.* (2004: iii) note: 'The hard slog of realist synthesis is about building up a picture of how various combinations of such contexts and circumstance can amplify or mute the fidelity of the intervention theory' (p. iii). Moreover, as Clegg (2005) argues, thinking from a critical realist perspective liberates the space for theoretically informed work, whereby arguments about method, and in particular RCTs, do not become a proxy for the open examination of ontological and epistemological assumptions. One of the underlying themes in critical realism is that of critique and emancipation, and evidence properly understood aligned to clear theoretical argumentation is part of this project. We claim that with its insistence that context is critical and that agents interact with and adapt to policies and interventions, realist synthesis is sensitive to diversity and change in program delivery and development.

The critical realist perspective recognizes the usefulness of research data generated by positivist-influenced, experimental designs, but only insofar as such data meet the requirements of real practice and policy questions in real contexts. From a critical realist perspective, findings from experimental studies can be combined with qualitative findings as both can help to refine the generative mechanism. For example, Pawson (2006) takes a critical realist approach in examining a practice question about the nature of the relationship between mentors and mentees in youth mentoring schemes. He begins with the presentation of a theoretical model and then analyzes a number of diverse and selectively chosen research studies in turn. Each study provides some insights that enhance the understanding of the theoretical model on mentoring. The process of research synthesis is theory driven, building on existing knowledge with new information and culminates in a more sophisticated model of youth mentoring relationships that is informed by research evidence. A pragmatic approach is evident in this process, as research studies are chosen for their relevance and usefulness to the practice issue of concern. The political context of practice is also acknowledged as a contested terrain in which evidence is negotiated and used to influence decision-making. The analysis of youth mentoring is in terms of what is occurring in the real world of social systems, institutions, resourcing and social values. Interpretive elements are also evident in the critical realistic perspective, which is sensitive to diversity, change and the requirements of different contexts of practice. The critical realistic approach is an example of how the four perspectives on evidence-based practice have been drawn together into an evolved hybrid approach to evidence-based practice that challenges the exclusivity of the positivist, scientific model.

Conclusion

This chapter has presented four theoretical perspectives that have influenced evidence-based practice, as it has been conceived and shaped within the social work profession. We have shown that no one theoretical approach to evidence-based social work – positivist, pragmatist, political or postmodern – can lay claim to being more ethical, more critically reflective or less authoritative. Evidence from RCTs, as from any other source, can be used in a narrow, authority-based way to support favoured practices or in a critically reflective, ethical way that acknowledges uncertainties and limitations, while questioning accepted practices. Likewise, qualitative and interpretive evidence, including practice wisdom, can be used in a narrow, authoritative way or in a critically reflective and ethical way. It is proposed that critical and ethical analysis is a fundamental feature of good evidence-based social work, which can incorporate a range of theoretical approaches to the production and use of evidence (Gray and McDonald 2006).

Evidence-based social work relies on the production and dissemination of evidence. If evidence-based social work were to develop into more than a debate between differing theoretical camps, there would be a need to generate research findings about the outcomes and effectiveness of a wide range of social work practices. Quality research studies that use a range of methodologies would be needed to add to the body of findings that are relevant and useful to practitioners in a range of contexts – useful both to the quality of practice and to the status of the profession. Evidence-based social work, however, involves more than the production of research findings. It requires that social workers take a critical stance in relation to their own practice and develop and use skills in critical analysis and research appraisal. It relies on the dissemination of findings to policy-makers, funding bodies, managers and social workers. It also relies upon the language, values, goals and theoretical understanding of evidence-based social work being incorporated into social work education and practice settings. The next two chapters examine the ways in which evidence-based practice has become incorporated into social work in various international contexts, with Chapter 4 focusing on global networks with a particular emphasis on the USA, and Chapter 5 dealing explicitly with the UK.

In conclusion, evidence-based practice is making a significant contribution to the framing of knowledge in social work, but evident in this activity is a struggle to *create a difference* between an inside expert specialty – in which social work researchers and practitioners can work – and an outside mixture of tensions and contradictory interests that cut through the specialty. There are tensions surrounding the extent of the social work evidence network, and conflict about what will stay inside and what will fall through the mesh. What is most significant in this process is how and who defines what constitutes knowledge in social work. Is knowledge primarily about information and skills, or is it the product of different theoretical perspectives, as described in this chapter, or is it the result of relationships and critical exchanges?

As will be discussed in detail in Chapter 5, some agencies and organizations in the UK, for example SCIE and the General Social Care Council, have recently attempted to capture what this knowledge is in social work. However, what is called 'knowledge' cannot be defined without an understanding of what 'gaining knowledge' means (Latour 1987). In other words, 'knowledge' is not something that can be described by itself or in opposition to 'ignorance' or 'opinion' but only by considering the entire cycle of accumulation through various network pathways. The key questions here are: how is knowledge rendered *mobile*, so that it can be retrieved or brought back; how is it kept *stable*, so it can be moved back and forth without distortion, corruption or decay; and how is it *combinable*, so that whatever stuff it is made of can be aggregated, or shuffled around like a pack of cards. As we show in the following chapters, evidence-based practice is one significant instance of this process at work in social work. We show how evidence-based practice, when translated into social work, constitutes an actor network, that is, as a socio-technical program it is dependent on a process of formalization whereby systems development and networks are central in legitimating the research program. The diffusion of evidence-based practice into social work takes the shape of a translation process with specific authorities of delimitation, which become the major vehicle that names, designates, mobilizes and formalizes evidence as an object for practice. The way in which the evidence-based network in social work gets formed depends on the mobility of actors and organizations and their ability to shift between roles and relations.

4 Globalizing the evidence

In this chapter, we examine the global diffusion of evidence-based practice (EBP) beginning with its development in the USA and continuing with its translation to international contexts. The theory of technology diffusion and adoption, as well as actor network theory used in Chapter 5, arise from the field of science and technology studies (STS). Beginning in the 1960s, diffusion theory seeks to explain the way in which technology is transferred and communicated outwards through social systems – or networks – in the belief that it is only a matter of time before it is adopted. The pace of diffusion is said to depend upon the innovation's perceived advantages, compatibility and comprehensibility, as well as the efficiency of the communication channels and information technology. Actor network theory, however, challenges the idea that innovations, such as evidence-based practice, and the technologies which support it, are stable entities that are passed from person to person – or group to group – through a process of *diffusion*. In diffusion theory, technologies are seen as independent of the different people – or systems – between which they are transferred. By way of contrast, actor network theory, influenced by Foucault's relational perspective linking space and networks, sees technology – machines – as an important actor or actant in a network, which, through a process of *translation* by actors, is either sustained or challenged by the network. It studies how networks evolve, how actors become enrolled (or do not) in processes and make alliances (or do not) with other actors in an attempt to ensure that particular depictions of 'progress' prevail (Davies 2002: 196). Both theories offer analytical frameworks for studying the way in which evidence-based practice arises and is adopted – or is not – by the social work fraternity. And they complement one another in the sense that actor network theory adds to diffusion theory explanations of the communication channels that enhance or obstruct translation, or diffusion and adoption, as the case may be. In other words, actor network theory seeks to show how pivotal actors – and nodes of networks – 'make sense' or 'nonsense' – of a new innovation in the process of promoting or obstructing its translation into practice.

As we shall see, there is much that proponents or innovators – i.e., the risk-takers and pioneers of evidence-based practice – can learn from diffusion theory. What is lacking in the push towards evidence-based practice in the case studies presented below is a coordinated, well-considered strategy to ensure its widespread adoption.

However, what is required is a twin-edged sword since a thorough and vigorous approach to persuade or convince social workers to abandon folklore approaches for systematic, scientific alternatives is likely to smack of social or systems engineering (Timmermans and Berg 2003). But the truth is that what is needed is 'a systematic, prescriptive model of adoption and diffusion' (Surry 1997).

What is missing thus far from the equation is any concerted attempt to focus on the wants and needs of the implementers, i.e., frontline social work practitioners. Heinz Kindler (2008: 322) makes this point succinctly in relation to the development of usable guidelines for child protection workers in Germany when he says that it is essential 'to stay in touch with frontline workers and families because *their needs legitimize our work*' (emphasis added). In the language of diffusion theory, what is needed is a pedagogically sound and technically advanced product that frontline practitioners would want to use and an effective and efficient means of teaching them how to use it. Much more attention needs to be paid to the challenge of utilization. Up until now, the focus has been on the proponents of evidence-based practice and on generating a literature which makes sense to academics and their students, with the result that, for most frontline practitioners, evidence-based practice remains 'academic'. From diffusion theory we learn that adopter-based approaches are inherently instrumental, with an eye to the end user who will ultimately implement the innovation in the practice setting *without taking them into account* in its development and diffusion. Academics go to conferences and run workshops for fellow academics and researchers on evidence-based practice – on how to conduct systematic reviews and meta-analyses. They also cement the idea at a macro level in trying to influence decision-makers, but little has been done at the micro level of the practice coalface. In this way, they defeat their own purposes, for the gap between theory and practice becomes an unbridgeable chasm. Hence the time has come for translation and implementation, which has already begun to receive attention in the USA and, to a lesser extent, in the UK and Canada. Haluk Soydan organized the 'First International Conference on Social Work and Translational Research' in Stockholm in October 2007, the proceedings of which will be published in the summer issue of *Research on Social Work Practice* in 2009.

Evidence-based practice exists and will only succeed within a social and professional context which *engages* with the real world of practice. As Tenner (1996: 9) notes, 'new structures, devices, and organisms react with real people in real situations in ways we could not foresee'. Until we can foresee them – until we can anticipate the consequences for practitioners at the coalface – our efforts will remain purely academic and will continue to meet with forceful resistance. The only way to increase the adoption of evidence-based practice is to engage with practitioners. Without a thorough understanding of the social system into which evidence-based practice is being introduced (Rogers 1995), no amount of resources – no matter how effectively and eloquently the principles of evidence-based practice are communicated or how efficient the communication channels – will enhance its uptake. Nor even will teaching it at university level, for new graduates all too easily become acculturated into the organizations in which they work, which are notoriously resistant to change. Once we have reviewed the case studies, the chapter ends with a brief discussion of Callon and Law's (1982) little-used local–global network framework to assess the global mobilization and uptake of evidence-based practice.

USA

The transferability of evidence-based practice to agency-based social work intervention in the USA remains a challenge, despite the growing evidence-base practice infrastructure (Gambrill 2006b; Mullen and Bacon 2004; Mullen, Bellamy *et al.* 2005). Thus Mullen, Bellamy *et al.* (2005: 63) referred to it as merely an 'idea about how practice might develop'. It is, therefore, erroneous to refer to it as a movement until global coordination is achieved. Nevertheless, evidence-based practice in the USA has advanced on a number of fronts. First, several education programs have introduced evidence-based practice into their graduate social work curriculum, mostly through the dedicated effort of key innovators at certain universities, e.g., Ed Mullen at Columbia, Karen Sowers at Tennessee, Stephanie Baus at Tulane, Stan McCracken at Chicago, and Bruce Thyer, when at Georgia, Aron Shlonsky at Toronto, and Aaron Rosen, David Pollio, Curtis McMillen, Enola Proctor and others at the George Warren Brown School of Social Work at Washington University. On this front, it would seem that the evidence-based practice lobby is making some inroads given consequent (i) requirements on students to conduct assignments using an evidence-based practice approach, and (ii) proliferation of literature on evidence-based practice, which has advanced the standing of certain key academics in the USA – and internationally – on both sides of the debate.

Second, a range of organizations, such as the Society for Social Work and Research (see below), have consistently promoted social work research, largely through agenda-setting activities at the annual program meetings of the Council of Social Work Education (CSWE)[1] – the peak social work education body in the USA. These formal networks constitute a growing interlocking evidence-based practice infrastructure that is steering social work in this direction at the macro level. Evidence-based practice is certainly the first perspective to develop into a coordinated effort at changing the field.

Third, the evidence-based practice bureaucracy, such as the Cochrane and Campbell Collaborations and the growing number of government-run clearing-houses, is generating SRs in areas related or tangential to social work practice, such as criminal justice and probation, child welfare – especially child protection – and education (see Chapter 2). As we shall see, the Social Welfare Coordinating Group of the Campbell Collaboration has experienced some difficulty in getting social workers to conduct SRs. Nevertheless, while in eight years of its existence, due mainly to a lack of time, motivation and skill, at the time of writing only twenty-one reviews have been completed, as well as twenty approved protocols and thirty-three titles in the field of social welfare, this compares favourably to the five completed reviews from the Education Group and the fourteen from the

Crime and Justice Group, indeed making it the most productive of the three groups within the Campbell Collaboration.

There is, however, development on another front, which is often confused with or wrongly assumed to constitute evidence-based practice, i.e., the empirically supported interventions (or treatments) approach (ESI/EST), pioneered by the Division 12 Task Force of the American Psychological Association (APA). US social work continues to draw quite heavily on this intervention effectiveness research. This has generated some disagreement within social work as to whether its ESI approach is indeed evidence-based practice, as we shall see.

US social workers' defensiveness about research for practice makes for a hard battle ahead, unless, as in education – where the 'No Child Left Behind' policy insists on SRs of practice using randomized controlled trials (RCTs) – it is written into social policy. This was the result of the efforts of a strong evidence-based practice lobby in education, in which the first Chair of the Campbell Collaboration, Robert Boruch, from the University of Pennsylvania, Graduate School of Education, had a hand.

Hence another front is that of evidence-based policy. Several US states require evidence-based interventions in certain fields (Corcoran 2007). Zlotnik (2007) notes that national bodies are following state examples: the National Association of Public Child Welfare Administrators (NAPCWA) has consequently developed the *Guide for child welfare administrators on evidence based practice* (2005). Policy-makers' interests in programs that are evidence based has led the state of California to support the California Evidence-Based Clearinghouse for Child Welfare[2] to consider the nature of evidence to guide child welfare practice. Hence there are signs that evidence-based policy is beginning to bite into the autonomy of professionals as to how and whether they should apply evidence. Zlotnik (2007: 627) believes that 'Teaching evidence-based child welfare practice and/or policy would help students understand that there is often a disconnect between policy intention and policy implementation and that funding, qualification and competencies of staff, and high caseloads are all factors affecting desired outcomes'. These are very real concerns.

It is important that we reflect on the more recent research-for-practice inno-vations beginning in the 1970s, in US social work, where three interweaving developments are discernible: (i) the researcher-practitioner initiative, (ii) the empirical-clinical practice initiative, and (iii) evidence-based practice. Loosely, we might say that these innovations spanned the 1980s, 1990s and 2000s respectively (see also Fischer 2009).

Research-for-practice

A defining moment in the research-for-practice or empirically based practice initiative, spurred on by a group of scholars – including Martin Bloom, Joel Fischer, Charles Glisson, Richard Grinnell and others – came with Joel Fischer's seminal piece published in 1973 entitled, 'Is casework effective?'. In reflecting on this, years later, Fischer thought that he had brought the social work profession to its knees (Fischer 2004). This is a marker for the beginning of more recent, concerted attempts to reduce the research–practice gap or rather to impress upon social workers the importance of researching the effectiveness of their practice (see also Fischer 1976, 1978a, 1978b; Jayaratne and Levy 1979; Mullen *et al.* 1972).

At the beginning of the 1970s, US casework theory, the dominant method of social work practice, was drawn together in Roberts and Nee's (1970) *Theories of social casework*. Much of practice was still heavily steeped in the Freudian-influenced diagnostic approach, which dates back to Mary Richmond's (1917) *Social diagnosis*. Its main opponent was the functional approach (Smalley, in Roberts and Nee 1970). In the year that Fischer's piece appeared, also published were Pincus and Minahan's (1973) universally acclaimed book, *Social work practice*, and for Goldstein's (1973) *Social work practice: a unitary approach*. There were signs of a distinct shift from social work's earlier connections with the medical professions to a systems approach, which sought to unite the diverse strands of social work. Ironically, with evidence-based practice thirty years later, the social work profession would again look to the medical profession for its dominant model. Nevertheless, the ecosystems perspective gained ground in the 1980s with the publication of Carol Germain and Alex Gitterman's (1980) *The life model of social work practice* and Carol Meyer's (1983) *Clinical social work in the ecosystems perspective*. Gambrill's (1983) *Casework: a competency-based approach* was also published at this time. On the fringes of this systems and eclectic influence in social work (Fischer 1978b), the push toward research on practice continued behind the scenes (Bloom and Gordon 1978). For the most part, then, social work was theoretically driven, or as Blythe and Briar (1985) noted, the models followed were largely theoretically rather than empirically based.

Through the 1980s, the researcher-practitioner – or 'scientific-practitioner' – model gained momentum (Bloom and Fischer 1982; Glisson and Fischer 1986; Thyer 1989; Grinnell 1988; Wakefield and Kirk 1996). As early as 1982, Bloom and Fischer were talking about evaluating practice as being crucial for professional *accountability*, following Briar (1973). Critics of this perspective wrongly accused its advocates of leaning too heavily on a behavioural approach, which, they claimed, was the most amenable to research (Bergin and Garfield (eds) 1971; Schwartz, in Rosenblatt and Waldvogel 1983; Thomas 1967; Wolpe 1969). However, there was a rich tradition of psychotherapy research predating the emergence of behaviour therapy (see Eysenck 1952). Even today, many texts on evidence-based practice (see for example Roberts and Yeager 2006) give the impression that social work is synonymous with psychotherapy (see Spiro 2007; Thyer 2007). The reliance of behavioural therapy, and psychotherapy in general, on research and success in conducting empirical outcome studies resides more in the philosophical assumptions of the approach, and its users' commitment to evaluation, rather than in the idea that the intervention or problems lent themselves more readily to research.

Following developments in psychotherapy, proponents advocated that prac-titioners measure change in client behaviour employing a single-system case design (Barlow and Hersen 1984; Blythe and Briar 1985; Mattaini 1996; Nelson, in

Grinnell 1988; Reid 1980; Ruckdeschel and Farris 1981). Others began developing clinical measurement instruments (Hudson 1982a, 1982b) and entreated social workers to familiarize themselves with statistics (Glisson and Fischer 1986) to enable them to research the effectiveness of their practice. Proponents of the research-for-and-on-practice approach attempted to make intervention more systematic by calling on practitioners to evaluate the effectiveness of their practice. Opponents lamented the positivist reductionism of the quantitative research approaches being advocated (Brekke 1986; Goldstein 1988; Heineman 1981; Heineman Pieper 1989; Imre 1984; Peile 1988; Ruckdeschel and Farris 1981; Weick 1987; Witkin and Gottschalk 1988). Yet, in fact, single-system designs were far more flexible than nomothetic research[3] designs, and even proponents of research-for-practice pointed to the undesirability of reductionism.

Fischer (1981) optimistically referred to these changes, including the development of single-case evaluation, as being somewhat revolutionary. He argued that 'a research technology [referring to the single-case design] that can be built into practice and can serve a number of functions that will enhance practice is now available to social workers. In and of itself, this development may be the highlight of – and certainly is a key to – the revolution in practice' (Fischer 1981: 201). This 'revolution' also reached the UK through the association between Brian Sheldon and Fischer (see Chapter 5). However, by the end of the 1980s, it became clear that this so-called 'revolution' had affected only a small part of social work in the USA (Penka and Kirk 1991) and the UK (Kazi and Wilson 1996).

Through the 1990s, the empirical-clinical practice approach – named after the title of Jayaratne and Levy's (1979) book – continued with proponents urging social workers to be more like researchers (Epstein 1996; Fischer 1993; Thyer 1991). But fierce opposition to the positivistic, quantitative research lobby in social work grew as opponents advocated for qualitative social work research approaches (Goldstein 1991; Kondrat 1992; Rodwell 1998; Ruckdeschel 1985; Tyson 1995; Witkin 1991). Many seminal texts on qualitative research had been published which were embraced by its advocates in social work (Denzin and Lincoln (eds) 1994; Lincoln and Guba 1985; Padgett 1998; Sherman and Reid 1994). Criticism continued as social workers resisted the rigid confines of what was required for empirically based practice. In 1996, a whole issue of *Social Work Research* [20(2)] was devoted to this debate and captured its fervour, showing no resolution in sight.

Though the evidence-based practice approach represents a complete break with these prior approaches, in that it is not so much about showing the after-the-fact effectiveness of individual instances – single cases – of practice as it is about anticipating interventions which might best be used for particular problems based on prior systematic effectiveness studies using SRs of RCTs, important precedents were set in this period. Hence the ambivalence with which social work educators and practitioners greeted evidence-based practice (Gray and McDonald 2006; Hall 2008; Witkin and Harrison 2001). Ed Mullen (2002: 6), another ardent promoter of evidence-based practice, in his reflection on the history of the research-for-practice 'movement' in social work, tells us that:

It was a short journey to the current embrace of evidence-based social work, but that journey would take the profession through a number of dead-end or, at least incomplete solutions such as *eclecticism, empiricism*, and the blending of science and practice in the *scientific-practitioner model* of social work. In addition, because the skepticism and search for pragmatic alternatives was occurring mostly in the social work research community and not in the practice community, a widening gap between practice and research grew to its current dimension, which is nothing short of a chasm.

In short, the empirical-clinical practice perspective entreated practitioners to base their practice on sound – concrete, empirical – research. While this effectiveness phase was labelled 'the age of performance accountability and program evaluation', many of the practice evaluations carried out at this time were deeply flawed, and often conducted internally with attendant bias towards positive evaluations.

Empirically supported interventions

A different innovation, coming out of clinical psychology, has further muddied the waters for evidence-based practice (Rubin 2008; Shlonsky forthcoming; Thyer 2008). As already outlined in Chapter 1, there is strong disagreement between advocates of evidence-based practice in social work, such as Bruce Thyer and Allen Rubin, and the credibility of ESIs as evidence-based practices in the plural, as Kevin Corcoran (2007) refers to them. ESIs have been variously referred to as 'empirically supported treatments' (Balas and Boren 2000; Bellamy *et al*. 2006; Bledsloe *et al*. 2007; Gibbs and Gambrill 2002; Mullen and Bacon 2004; Mullen, Shlonsky *et al*. 2005; Weissman and Sanderson 2001) and 'evidence-based psychotherapies' (Bledsloe *et al*. 2007; Weissman *et al*. 2006). As already mentioned, empirically supported treatments originated from the APA Division 12 Task Force, organized in the early 1990s to promote and disseminate information for both the practitioner and the general public on the random-assignment, controlled-outcome study literature of psychotherapy, psychoactive medications and psychological procedures. The Task Force's purpose was to develop evidentiary standards to be used to designate a given treatment or assessment method as 'empirically validated' – later changed to 'empirically supported' – and to *review the literature* and publish lists of treatments that met or did not meet these evidentiary standards. The Task Force established two sets of standards or evidence benchmarks, one to designate an intervention as 'empirically supported' (hence ESTs) or 'well supported', and another, less stringent one, used to designate an intervention as 'promising' or 'probably efficacious'. Two major publication pathways emerged from the Task Force's efforts to compile these lists of 'approved' treatments: an edited collection by Nathan and Gorman (2007), *A guide to treatments that work* (3rd edn) and a series of online articles[4] to which nothing new has been added since 1998. A new Division 12 developed, edited and supported a book series entitled Keeping Up with the Advances in Psychotherapy: Evidence-based Practice, published by Hogrefe and Huber. Note the crucial terminology change from 'empirically supported' to 'evidence-based', because the criteria for the two are entirely differ-ent. The EST approach continues through the efforts of the Committee on Science and Practice, Society of Clinical Psychology (e.g., Section III of Division 12 of the APA), chaired by David Klonsky, PhD. However, according to Thyer (2008), it has been overtaken by evidence-based practice.

Allen Rubin (2008: 6) is critical of ESIs, which are only called 'evidence based' if the practitioner is providing a specific intervention that appears on the list of interventions (see Weissman *et al.* 2006) 'whose effectiveness has been supported by a sufficient number of rigorous experimental outcome evaluations to merit their "seal of approval" as an evidence-based intervention'. For Rubin and Parrish (2007a), evidence-based practice involves a combination of the 'proc-ess perspective' that leads to locating and appraising credible evidence as part of the evidence-based practice decision-making approach as well as the 'interven-tion perspective' emphasized by ESIs. Importantly, managed care companies and other influential sources are promoting ESIs and, in the process, distorting evidence-based practice when they define it merely as 'a list of what intervention to use automatically for what diagnosis, regardless of ... professional expertise and special understanding of idiosyncratic client characteristics and circum-stances' (Rubin 2008: 6). Sackett *et al.*'s (2000) revised definition incorporates practitioner judgement and client values and preferences (Barber, in White 2008; Rubin 2008; Rubin and Babbie 2008) and is 'consistent with the scientific method, which holds that all knowledge is provisional and subject to refutation' (Rubin 2008: 7).

As with all initiatives to promote the use of research for practice, there is a considerable gap between the availability of ESTs and their uptake by social workers (Balas and Boren 2000; Bellamy *et al.* 2006; Brekke *et al.* 2007; Gibbs and Gambrill 2002; Mullen and Bacon 2004; New York State Office of Mental Health 2001; Soydan 2007). Bledsloe *et al.* (2007) identified a lack of training in ESIs as a key barrier to their use by social work practitioners (Bellamy *et al.* 2006; Mullen, Shlonsky *et al.* 2005; New Freedom Commission on Mental Health 2003; Weissman and Sanderson 2001). Bledsloe *et al.* (2007) reported that findings from a recent dissemination and implementation project support the need for prior train-ing in ESTs for social workers to implement them in practice (see also Bellamy *et al.* 2006; Bledsoe *et al.* 2007).

Weissman *et al.* (2006) conducted a national survey of social work training programs in psychotherapy, noting that clinical social workers were the largest providers of mental health services in the USA, and found more than 50 per cent wanting in 'gold standard'-defined psychotherapy training, i.e., didactic training and clinical supervision. Weissman *et al.* (2006: 6–7) defined evidence-based psychotherapies – equated with ESTs – as comprising:

... at least two randomized controlled trials of a manual-defined treatment. In classifying treatment as [EST] we also required that the trials have samples of sufficient power, with well characterized patients with specific psychiat-ric disorders, with randomly assigned control conditions of psychotherapy, placebo, pill or other treatment and with at least two different investigative teams demonstrating efficacy.

Note that evidence-based practice has no such specifications as to the number of RCTs it takes to validate a treatment nor does it advocate specific treatments for particular populations. It relies heavily on a chain of factors – best available evidence, the practitioner's judgement and the patient's needs – and not simply on the proven effectiveness of particular interventions. Practitioners employing the ESI approach rely heavily on the Division 12 Task Force on Psychological Interventions' list of efficacious, empirically supported psychological treatments for specific populations. It defines a 'well-established psychotherapy' in one of two ways:

1   Having at least two good between-group design experiments that must demonstrate efficacy in one or more of the following ways:

    (i)   superiority to pill or psychotherapy placebo or to other treatment, and
    (ii) equivalence to already established treatment with adequate sample sizes.

2   Supported by a large series of single-case design experiments demonstrating efficacy with

    (i)   the use of good experimental design, and
    (ii) comparison of the intervention with another treatment. (Chambless *et al.* 1998)

Using either of these initial criteria, experiments must also be conducted with treatment manuals or equivalent clear descriptions of treatment; characteristics of samples must be specified; and effects must be demonstrated by at least two different investigators or teams (Chambless *et al.* 1998). 'Probably efficacious treatments' are defined in one of three ways:

1   Two experiments that show the treatment is superior to a waiting-list control group.
2   One or more experiments that meet all well-established criteria with the exception of requiring effects being demonstrated by two different investigators or teams.
3   A small series of single-case design experiments that must meet well-established treatment criteria. (Chambless *et al.* 1998)

The list of ESTs or so-called 'evidence-based therapies' identified by Weismann *et al.* (2006) using the above criteria 'blackboxes' psychotherapies by implying that there is sound evidence that these treatments work – or that they do not, as the case may be – without citing the RCT studies to support this selection. Furthermore, the list provides ammunition for the strong psychodynamic lobby, which still predominates in the USA and for whom intrapsychic processes – such as defence mechanisms, transferential dynamics, unconscious transactions and ego functions, as well as attachment theory, the psychology of self, relational theory and, of course, psychodynamic theory – continue to undergird clinical social work. For psychodynamic theorists, the client–worker relationship is central. Hence they often point to the scant evidence that particular interventions contribute to positive outcomes over and above factors such as the client–therapist relationship and the personality of the psychotherapist (e.g., Chambless 2002; Drisko 2004; Reid 1997; Thyer 2007; Wampold 2001). However, there is mounting scientific evidence showing that practitioner effectiveness is influenced by relationship factors *as well as* the type of intervention employed (Besa 1994; Cody 1991; Reid 1997; Roseborough 2006; Rubin 2007a; Thyer 2007). Psychodynamic clinicians would also do well to pay attention to research on the effectiveness of psychoanalytic treatment (see, for example, De La Parra and Del Rio 2005; Erle and Goldberg 2003; Fonagy (ed.) 2002; Sandell *et al.* 2000).

For behavioural practitioners, the interdisciplinary Council for Training in Evidence-Based Behavioral Practice (EBBP), sponsored by the National Institutes of Health's Office of Behavioral and Social Science Research (OBSSR),[5] recently began to offer online training modules on the EBBP process, searching for evidence and systematic reviews. These online training courses are designed to help behavioural practitioners and students to acquire tools that integrate research and practice in real-world conditions. The 'EBBP Process' module aims to enhance the skills of behavioural interventionists from a variety of healthcare disciplines to find, appraise and apply evidence to improve the health of individuals, communities and other populations. In 'Searching for Evidence', behavioural health professionals learn about available online resources and develop skills to search for healthcare evidence. In 'Systematic Reviews', evidence users learn to appraise the quality of systematic reviews and evidence creators learn the basic steps in conducting a systematic review. Instructors who use the modules or other EBBP materials in their courses are also invited to share syllabi, conference presentations and other resources in the new EBBP Teaching Resource Library.[6] EBBP.org training materials are based on an analysis of the professional competencies required to engage in the EBBP process. The EBBP Council white paper[7] describing these competencies was compiled by an interdisciplinary group of Council members representing the disciplines of medicine, nursing, psychology, social work, public health and information sciences. The result is a harmonized approach to the evidence-based practice process across the major professions delivering behavioural interventions.

Whether or not the researcher-practitioner, empirical-clinical practice and ESI approaches are precursors of or part of the development of evidence-based practice remains the subject of ongoing debate. But, as Eileen Gambrill, Bruce Thyer, Allen Rubin and others continue to emphasize, the definitions of each are entirely different. Further, the list of ESTs, similar to that cited by Weisman *et al.* (2006), is vague, erroneous and misleading.

Evidence-based practice

In prior chapters we have discussed the nature of the evidence-based practice approach. In this chapter, we are concerned with the way in which this approach has been translated and adopted within social work. Important to the process of diffusion or translation is the development of an infrastructure for the promulgation and transfer of an innovation within and between contexts. What prior initiatives in the research-for-practice movement lacked was the benefit of information technology. However, we learn from diffusion theory that technology, by itself, does not bring about change. As MacKenzie (1996: 7) notes, the best products are not always the ones people want to use, and the same might be said about the 'best available evidence', no matter how well it is communicated: 'Technologies … may be best because they have triumphed, rather than triumphing because they are best'. In other words, the key lies in being able to convince practitioners to use the evidence-based practice approach.

Everett M. Rogers, the pioneer of diffusion theory, in his theory of perceived attributes (Rogers 1995), advanced the idea that adopters judge an innovation based on their perceptions of its trialability, observability, relative advantage, complexity and compatibility (with their current work practices). This theory holds that an innovation's diffusability – or transferability – is enhanced if it (i) can be tried on a limited basis before it is adopted – a 'use before you buy' approach; (ii) offers observable or tangible results or benefits; (iii) has an advantage over other innovations or existing practices – the status quo; (iv) is not too complex; and (v) is compatible with existing practices and values. It is here, however, that evidence-based practice reaches a sticking point.

Many social workers see technology as dehumanizing, a device which distances them from clients. They also fear a loss of autonomy when the tools of technology replace the humanistic aspects of their practice. Thus claims that an innovation will maximize efficiency and effectiveness and eliminate error are likely to fall on deaf ears until a user-oriented approach is adopted. Burkman's (1987) product utilization theory rejects the idea that technological superiority is all that is needed to convince people to adopt an innovation. He advocates a program of 'user-oriented instructional development' in which innovators identify potential adopters and take time to understand their perceptions of – and objections to – an innovation. Even better, end users could be involved in the process of 'innovation development' to ensure a user-friendly product. Once instruction has been provided in the use of the innovation, it is essential that post-adoption support is provided. Up until now this has not been the approach within evidence-based practice, where most of the effort has been focused on the macro – infrastructure – level, which includes the generation of 'gold standard' research and systematic reviews, rather than the micro – end user – level.

As we shall see in Chapter 5, the evidence-based practice infrastructure for social care in the UK appears better developed than that in the USA, though certain peak bodies, like the National Institute for Mental Health (NIMH) appear to be changing that. Perhaps the most long-established advocate of evidence-based practice in US social work is the Society for Social Work and Research (SSWR).

Organizing the evidence-based practice infrastructure

As we shall see from the discussion which follows, organizations promoting research in social work in the USA have formed a close-knit network which is fast becoming the first coordinated effort – at an organizational level – within US social work to change the face of education and practice.

The Society for Social Work and Research

Founded in 1994 by Janet Williams, with strong support from Bruce Thyer, the Society for Social Work and Research (SSWR), as its name suggests, is dedicated to the advancement of social work research and strongly promotes evidence-based practice. According to its website (www.sswr.org), it has over 1,200 members – drawn from more than 200 universities and institutions across the world – from forty-five states in the USA as well as from Denmark, Hong Kong, Israel and the UK. The current president is Sarah Gehlert. Former presidents include founder Williams, Tony Tripodi, Allen Rubin, Nancy Hooyman, Paula Allen-Meares, Deborah Padgett and Anne Fortune, all of whom have been consistent proponents of social work research. Sage's journal *Research on Social Work Practice*, edited by Bruce Thyer, which publishes empirical work in social work, is part of SSWR members' subscription benefits and SSWR's website also has a link to Sage's *Qualitative Social Work* journal, which publishes debates and papers on qualitative social work research, of which Roy Ruckdeschel is joint editor with Ian Shaw in the UK.

SSWR maintains links with several social work and research-focused organizations in the USA, including the National Institutes for Health (NIH), particularly the National Institute of Mental Health (NIMH) – which played a large part in SSWR's establishment by funding a landmark report compiled by David M. Austin (1991) – and the Institute for the Advancement of Social Work Research (IASWR), which plays a national advocacy role (see also Austin 1992, 1999; Rubin 2007c). In fact, there is a strong network of organizations aiming to promote social work research which is beginning to build the US evidence-based practice infrastructure. It includes the Action Network for Social Work Education and Research (ANSWER), which is another SSWR partner.

Action Network for Social Work Education and Research

The Action Network for Social Work Education and Research (ANSWER)[8] is a coalition whose mission is to increase legislative and executive branch advocacy on behalf of social work education, training and research. It accomplishes its mission through collaboration among social work education, research and practice organizations; social work education programs; and other interest groups. Member organizations include the Association of Baccalaureate Social Work Program Directors (BPD), Council on Social Work Education (CSWE), Institute for the Advancement of Social Work Research (IASWR), Group for the Advancement of Doctoral Education (GADE), National Association of Deans and Directors of Schools of Social Work (NADD), National Association of Social Workers (NASW), and the SSWR.

Consortium of Social Science Associations

SSWR also has links to the Consortium of Social Science Associations (COSSA), a US advocacy organization that promotes attention to and federal funding for the social and behavioural sciences. It serves as a bridge between academic research and the Washington policy-making community. Its members include more than 100 professional associations, scientific societies, universities and research centres and institutes. Padgett (2005: 4) describes COSSA as 'a watchdog group that keeps its members informed and advocates on their behalf for research funding and in opposing political interference in scientific research'. She goes on to say that 'Recent attacks on National Institutes of Health-funded (NIH) studies by some right-wing legislators have rendered COSSA ever more important' (*ibid.*).

Internationally SSWR has co-sponsored the International Conference on Evaluation for Practice[9] and is an active participant in the Campbell Collaboration. The SSWR has been lobbying for some time to establish a National Center for Social Work Research[10] but has, as yet, been unsuccessful in this endeavour (see Rubin 2007b). Padgett (2005: 6–7) lists SSWR's objectives as being to:

1   encourage scientific rigour even as we embrace the use of multiple methods – quantitative, qualitative, and mixed – to address the complex social problems we seek to understand and ameliorate;
2   be on the leading edge of fostering and disseminating intervention and evaluation research and the theory development that guides these efforts;
3   maintain and build our support for students and early-career scholars;
4   maintain and expand our partnerships with other social work organizations and other professional societies in advocating for independent inquiry and socially and ethically responsible research;
5   encourage international colleagues to participate in SSWR and at our annual conference since cross-national collaboration is beneficial to all concerned with the promotion of social work and social work research worldwide.

However, there is little evidence of evidence-based social work research – based on RCTs and SRs – on the SSWR website. The organization appears to play an advocacy rather than a research role, though it has run methodology workshops, including qualitative and mixed-methods research and intervention research (Padgett 2005: 6). It has focused its efforts on the generators rather than the end users of evidence.

Institute for the Advancement of Social Work Research

While SSWR is an organization of individual members committed to advancing quality social work research and scholarship, IASWR is composed of the major social work leadership organizations: the Council on Social Work Education (CSWE), the National Association of Social Workers (NASW), National Association of Deans and Directors (NADD), the Association of Baccalaureate Program Directors (BPD), and the Group for the Advancement of Doctoral Education (GADE). It works at a national level to create and strengthen the resources through federal and foundation funding, such as the NIMH Social Work Research Development Centres, the NIDA development centres, and the CDC funding. IASWR also sponsors technical assistance workshops. The current president is Joan Zlotnik.

In conjunction with NIMH, the IAWSR has developed a comprehensive document on *Partnerships to Integrate Evidence-Based Mental Health Practices into Social Work Education and Research* (2007). This is a significant development, given that the majority of social work practitioners in the US work within the field of mental health. It has also conducted a systematic review of research on the retention of child welfare workers, which failed to produce any 'strong' evidence due to the lack of consistency across studies (Zlotnik 2007; Zlotnik *et al.* 2005).

There thus appears to be a close network of organizations in the USA working to promote social work – and social science – research and evidence-based practice. While there is some alignment of organizational objectives, there is, too, competition for resources. What is needed is a united coalition for evidence-based practice, rather than a network of organizations sharing a common goal.

The Campbell Collaboration

While these bodies have been influential in promoting social work research, evidence-based practice remains weak in social work. Nevertheless there have been certain key events in nudging US social work towards evidence-based practice as it is practised within medicine where it originated. One such event was a meeting held in London in July 1999, where eighty participants from five countries gathered to explore the idea of developing a similar body to Cochrane for the social sciences (see Chapter 5). At this meeting, a steering group was formed, as well as discussion groups to represent the interests of the participating professions – namely, criminal justice and probation, education, and social work and social care – grouped as social welfare and hereafter referred to as the Social Welfare Coordinating Group (SWCG). For social workers, the SWCG was pivotal, with Haluk Soydan – then from the Centre for Evaluation of Social Services under the Swedish National Board of Health and Welfare in Stockholm and now at the University of Southern California – the initial leader of this group. He was also appointed to the Campbell Steering Group. Another key player early in the process from social work and member of the planning group was Geraldine Macdonald who, as we shall see in Chapter 5, was instrumental in the development of evidence-based social work in the UK. Other participants from social work included Ron Feldman from Columbia

University, Ian Sinclair from York University in the UK, and Neil Weiner, Ira Schwartz and Lawrence Sherman from the University of Pennsylvania.

At the beginning of 2000, when the Campbell Collaboration – or C2 as it became known by many of its members – was formally established, Dorothy de Moya was hired as *pro bono* secretary and played an important role in the continuity of its work until its first full-time executive director took office in 2005. At the inaugural meeting in February 2000, C2 established its base at the University of Pennsylvania under the leadership of Robert Boruch, from the Graduate School of Education. At this meeting, a Review Group on social work and social welfare was formed with subgroups (and chairs) for Child Welfare (John Schuerman), Housing and Transportation (Mark Petticrew), Child Development and Learning Disabilities (Geraldine Macdonald), and Immigration and Ethnic Issues (Haluk Soydan). A further key event for social work was a meeting which followed in Atlanta in the USA, where members of the Campbell SWCG (John Schuerman, Haluk Soydan and others) met with the SSWR in January 2001. At this meeting, an alliance between the SSWR and Campbell Collaboration was forged and evidence-based practice in social work in the USA was born.

The First Annual Campbell Collaboration Colloquium was held at the University of Pennsylvania in February 2001. It was attended by 150 participants. The program included a review of the progress of C2's first year, an examination of methodological issues involved in conducting C2 systematic reviews and presentations on issues pertaining to literature searching, publication bias, study coding, coding reliability, and statistical issues important to conducting useful meta-analytic reviews of the type that C2 encourages. Appropriate methods for including the findings of qualitative studies and process evaluations in systematic reviews were also examined. The conference was addressed by John DiIulio, President G.W. Bush's then nominee for Director, White House Office of Faith-Based and Community Initiatives, examining 'What Works in Delivering Government Services: Faith-Based or Not'. DiIulio emphasized that all social interventions – those which were faith-based and otherwise – should be subjected to scientific scrutiny. The SWCG did not publish systematic reviews during the first year of C2 and Mark Petticrew became group chair (SSWR Newsletter, December 2001: 12).

In 2002 Bruce Thyer was elected to serve as SSWR's liaison with C2, which, at the time, was co-chaired by Haluk Soydan, who was also co-chair of the SWCG with Geraldine Macdonald in the UK (see Chapter 5) at the time. In reporting on his attendance at the C2 board meeting in Baltimore in September 2002, Thyer noted that *systematic reviews*, unlike practice guidelines (and ESIs), did not tell practitioners what to do (or which interventions to use). They were summaries and conclusions drawn from scientifically credible research, not protocols for practice. Systematic reviews contribute to the development of evidence-based practice guidelines and draw the line at providing explicit directions for practitioners (SSWR Newsletter, November 2002: 7).

Julia Littell, SSWR representative to C2 in 2004, reported that evidence-based practice had increased the demand for empirical information on the effects of psychosocial interventions and social policies. She extolled the value of careful reviews and syntheses but noted the shortcomings of systematic reviews (see Chapter 2). With Arild Bjørndal, Littell was elected co-chair of the SWCG.

In 2004, C2 held its fifth annual colloquium in Lisbon, Portugal, which featured plenary presentations by policy-makers from around the world, a series of workshops on systematic review methods, and papers on research synthesis and the use of evidence in practice and policy. A new users group was formed to identify important questions for systematic reviews and to help translate results into formats that were easily accessible to a diverse audience.

In June 2005, C2 entered into an agreement with the American Institutes for Research (AIR) to leverage support for international efforts to inform and improve policy and practice. Under this agreement, C2 hired an executive director, founding member Dr Philip Davies, and three managing editors (one for each of the C2 substantive areas): Crime and Justice Group, David Wilson from George Mason University; SWCG, Julia Littell from Bryn Mawr College; Education, Herbert Turner from Pennsylvania. The new director, an academic with thirty years experience, hailed from the UK where he was director of social sciences in the Department for Continuing Education at Oxford University. He had served in the UK Cabinet Office, as deputy director of the Government Social Research Unit (GSRU) and the Economic and Social Research Council's Research Evaluation Committee. However, his tenure was very brief.

The sixth annual C2 colloquium was held in Los Angeles in February 2006, hosted by the University of Southern California (USC) School of Social Work, where Haluk Soydan is now based. It was co-sponsored by SSWR, IASWR, AIR and others. The colloquium was well attended by social work scholars and focused once again on the production of high-quality systematic reviews. USC and IASWR sponsored a briefing on C2 systematic reviews on Capitol Hill on 31 March 2006. The briefing highlighted C2 systematic reviews on anti-terrorism strategies, parent involvement in children's education, and the effects of mainstream programs for juvenile delinquency on majority and minority youth. Also in June 2006, IASWR, as part of its networking role, organized a series of meetings to introduce C2 to staff of the NIH Office of Behavioral and Social Science Research, US DHHS Office of the Assistant Secretary for Planning and Evaluation, and members of national professional and social science associations.

In June 2007, C2 ended its formal agreement with AIR and Phil Davies stepped down as C2 executive director, in order to continue his work at AIR. Arild Bjørndal was elected co-chair of the C2 Steering Group, replacing Haluk Soydan. The Steering Group formed *ad hoc* working groups to develop proposals for changes in C2 governance and communication, membership and voting rights, information systems and publications. Discussions were underway with publishers interested in publishing the C2 Library. C2 welcomed three new partner organizations: University of Toronto School of Social Work (Aron Shlonsky), York University in Toronto (David Phipps), and CanKnow (Phil Abrami).

Ways to increase systematic reviews included a proposed new Public Health Review Group, expanding the number of editors with expertise in specific fields of social welfare practice and peer reviewers, and actively soliciting systematic reviews. Also the Nordic Campbell Centre and others identified 'burning topics' for systematic reviews in social welfare, and existing research addressing those topics. The SWCG invited authors of prior reviews to consider 'Campbellizing' their reviews. Acknowledging that this might involve improvements in some aspects of the review process, the SWCG undertook to explore sources of funding for these reviews. It also issued a broad call for titles for systematic reviews in social welfare. The SWCG decided to move toward an elected leadership such that the group's co-chairs and steering group representatives would, in future, be elected by SWCG members.

C2 held its seventh annual colloquium in London in May 2007, where it was agreed that membership would be open to anyone who had ever attended a C2 SWCG meeting (at SSWR or previous C2 colloquia), authored a C2 SWCG review, or served as a peer reviewer for the SWCG. The meeting again featured plenary presentations by policy-makers from around the world, a series of workshops on systematic review methods, and papers on research synthesis and the use of evidence in practice and policy. SSWR members who presented papers and chaired sessions at this meeting included Judith Rycus, Aron Shlonsky, Joanne Yaffe and Joan Levy Zlotnik.

The C2 Steering Group accepted an offer of core support from the government of Norway for the second half of 2007 and for 2008–2010. In 2008, C2's head office moved to the Norwegian Knowledge Centre for the Health Services located in Oslo, Norway, with Mark Lipsey as Steering Group co-chair. Three new members joined the C2 SWCG, namely, Esther Coren (UK), Dennis Gorman (USA) and Sten Anttila (Sweden) along with recent additions, Paul Montgomery (UK), Bruce Thyer (USA) and Joanne Yaffe (USA). Priorities for organizational development included moving toward a more open, democratic organizational structure and increasing the production of relevant and rigorous systematic reviews. Julia Littell received a two-year grant of $61,000 from the Swedish Institute for Evidence-Based Social Work Practice to support her efforts to build the capacity of social work scholars to conduct rigorous systematic reviews of research on topics relevant for social work and social welfare.

The eighth annual C2 colloquium was held in Vancouver, Canada, in May 2008 hosted by a consortium of Canadian organizations, with support from AIR. Yet again the focus was on the use of systematic reviews in practice and policy. Many of the systematic reviews conducted by Campbell collaborators relate to contexts of social work practice, such as social welfare, child welfare or mental health or, in the case of ESIs, to psychotherapy. There have been no systematic reviews on the effectiveness of social work practice, although Rubin and Parrish (2007b) found twenty-eight published studies using RCTs in social work journals between 2000 and 2005 and, much earlier, Fischer (1973) had found seventeen. However, most social work research tends to be small-scale and localized, employing a mixed-methods or largely qualitative research approach (Shek *et al.* 2005). Hence, as outlined in Chapter 2, most social work research does not meet 'gold standard' Campbell criteria and would not be included in their systematic reviews.

After eight years in operation, the C2 SWCG, as already mentioned, has produced more reviews than the other two groups. Over the years, the main social work scholars who have been actively involved in C2 include Haluk Soydan (USC) who served as co-chair of the C2 Steering Group for many years, Eileen Gambrill (Berkeley), Ed Mullen (Columbia), Bruce Thyer (Florida State University), John Schuerman (Chicago) and, more recently, Aron Shlonsky.

Programming the evidence

The 'Road Ahead' report (US Department of Health and Human Services 2006: 17) asserts that 'currently, too few mental health graduate training programs devote adequate time to education on evidence-based methods of diagnosis, treatment, or evaluation'. According to Proctor (2007: 586):

> ... most providers cite graduate school as the source of their initial training in EBP ... But schools of social work are not mandated to provide training in EBP, and most schools do not disseminate EBPs or train practitioners for their use ... Thus, social work education shares culpability for the nation's insufficient supply of EBP-trained practitioners.

Hence an important focus of the evidence-based practice infrastructure has been social work education and the teaching of evidence-based practice (Howard *et al.* 2003; Shlonsky forthcoming, see also *Research on Social Work Practice* 17(5)). Another key event for advancing evidence-based practice in US social work was the first national conference – the National Symposium on Improving the Teaching of Evidence-Based Practice – convened by Allen Rubin at the University of Texas at Austin in October 2006. It involved over 200 participants from seventy universities. While mainly from the USA, a few participants came from Sweden (Haluk Soydan) and Canada (Aron Shlonsky). A selection of papers from this conference was published in the September 2007 issue of *Research on Social Work Practice* (volume 17(5)), guest edited by Allen Rubin, whose editorial seeks to synthesize the proceedings. Certainly a key factor in the development of evidence-based practice rests on creating a learning environment where evidence-based practice is encouraged and facilitated, i.e., where aspiring social workers are taught to use this approach. But, as already outlined, this is not sufficient without a simultaneous 'focus on the adoption of a specific innovation by a specific set of potential adopters' (Surry 1997: 5), namely, social work practitioners who supervise students in their agency placements. Instead the main focus has been on bolstering this educational force by generating a prolific amount of books and journal articles on evidence-based practice. Aron Shlonsky (forthcoming) has written most recently on the progress of evidence-based practice education in social work in the USA and has this to say:

> George Warren Brown University in St Louis was the first school to reshape its entire curriculum to reflect a 'practice guidelines' approach (Howard,

McMillen, and Pollio, 2003), including measures to insure that students are trained in at least one EST (e.g., cognitive behavioral therapy for depression). The University of Toronto [where Shlonsky is based] changed its approach to teaching research, opting to teach the steps of EBP and training students to evaluate research rather than training them to conduct research. Oxford University [in the UK, see Chapter 5] has gone in yet a different direction and, rather than offering a degree in social care, is now offering a degree in evidence-based social intervention. More recently, other schools have begun to reshape their approach to teaching social work. For instance, Columbia University is now offering several courses in EBP and has begun to shape its curriculum accordingly, and the University of Tennessee is now in the process of infusing their entire curriculum with EBP. Of course, there are others and an even larger number of individual academics who are integrating EBP into their courses [such as Riaan van Zyl at the University of Louisville in Kentucky, formerly from South Africa (see van Zyl, in Thyer and Kazi 2004)].

Shlonsky advocates problem-based learning, developed at McMaster University in Canada, as the approach of choice in teaching evidence-based practice to equip students with the requisite critical thinking skills and questioning approach it requires. Problem-based learning was pioneered in Australia by the medical school at the University of Newcastle, where the authors of this volume hail from. The approach was adapted by the social work department to an experience-based approach to reflect the strengths-based focus of social work (English *et al.* 1994; Gibbons and Gray 2002, 2004; Gray and Gibbons 2002; Plath *et al.* 1999). It was also an approach strongly advocated by Howard Goldstein (2001).

Within this pedagogical model, content – for example, on culturally competent practice, social work values, research, and ethical decision-making – is not taught in discrete courses but runs through each level of the curriculum (Gray and Gibbons 2007). Considerable time is spent in curriculum planning and review, and faculty work together closely as a team to share information about what is being taught across the curriculum. Also, related areas are taught together in learning units – for example, research, policy and ethics might be taught in a single unit (Gibbons and Gray 2005).

With the US case study, we see the beginnings of evidence-based practice in social work as marked by the establishment of the Campbell Collaboration even though there were precedents to evidence-based social work in its forerunners, the researcher-practitioner and empirical-clinical practice approaches and, more recently, the ESIs approach. Evidence-based social work seems to adopt a looser definition of evidence-based practice. It seems to be more mechanically focused around what Rubin (2008) calls the 'intervention perspective' and fails to suffi-ciently incorporate the *process* of evidence-based practice and its interacting core elements of practitioner expertise, client values and preferences and available best evidence. However, Mullen, Bellamy *et al.* (2005) see evidence-based social work and evidence-based practice in social work as synonymous. Gibbs (2003: 6) believes that what makes evidence-based social work unique is that it places clients first:

... evidence-based practitioners adopt a process of lifelong learning that involves continually posing questions of *direct practical importance to clients*, searching objectively and efficiently for the current best evidence relative to each question, and taking appropriate action guided by evidence [emphasis added].

What is common to these approaches is their attempt to get social workers to engage in 'research-based practice'; what separates them and makes evidence-based practice in social work distinct is the comprehensiveness of the evidence-based practice approach and its attempt to move social workers beyond using research or evaluating their own practice in the style of the empirical-clinical practitioner approach, to being able to locate and critically appraise empirical evidence (Gambrill 2003; Mullen, Bellamy *et al.* 2005). All this is being done without any concerted engagement with practitioners at the coalface.

Globalizing evidence

In this next section, we examine the way in which evidence-based practice has been diffused through international contexts where key US actors, such as Ed Mullen and Bruce Thyer, have played a leading role in its promotion. Perhaps the pivotal key player in this international context has been Haluk Soydan, who, we shall see, was a prime mover in the development of evidence-based practice in Sweden and continues his international promotion of evidence-based practice since his move to Southern California, most recently into China.

Europe (including Scandinavia)

In the European context, a key actor in the diffusion of practice evaluation research has been the Inter-Centre Network for the Evaluation of Social Work Practice (or Intsoceval).[11] The network developed as a consequence of the International Conference on Social Work and Evaluation Research, organized by Haluk Soydan in Stockholm in 1997, the proceedings of which were published in the *International Journal of Social Welfare* in 1998. It is a well-established network of research centres (see Table 4.1) which, since 1998, has held annual conferences hosted by member centres in different locations. Conference themes have included: The research-practice relationship (York 1998); Researcher-practitioner partnership and research implementation (Stockholm 1999); Outcome and measurement of outcome of social work intervention (Utrecht 2000); Evaluation as an instrument for knowledge-based social care (Helsinki 2001); International perspectives on social work knowledge (Stirling 2003); Evidence-based social work (Switzerland 2004); and Stakeholder participation in delivering evidence-based policy and practice (SCIE, London 2005). It is only in recent years that there has been a shift from practice evaluation to evidence-based practice by Intsoceval. However, there does not seem to be much evidence of its influence in the home countries of its member centres. With some exceptions – the Social Care Institute of Excellence

Table 4.1 Inter-Centre Network for the Evaluation of Social Work Practice[a]

Country	Research centre[b]	Key actor
Denmark	Research Unit of Social Work Practice, Danish University of Education	Inge Beryderup
England	Collaborative Research Group: Primary Care and Community Social Work, University of Sheffield	Peter Marsh
	Social Care Institute for Excellence (SCIE)	Mike Fisher
	Social Work Research and Development Unit (SWRDU), http://www.york.ac.uk/inst/swrdu/ Social Policy Research Unit (SPRU), http://www.york.ac.uk/inst/spru/ University of York	Ian Shaw
Finland	Finnish Evaluation of Social Services (FinSoc) National Research and Development Centre for Welfare and Health (STAKES), http://groups.stakes.fi/FINSOC/EN/index.htm	Riitta Haverinen
	University of Jyvaskyla	Mikko Mantysaari
Netherlands	Verwey-Jonker Institute for Research into Social Issues	Willem Melief
Scotland	University of Stirling	Gill McIvor
Sweden	Institute of Evidence-based Social Work Practice (IMS)	Knut Sundell
Switzerland	School of Social Work, Research and Development Department, University of Applied Sciences	Peter Sommerfeld
USA	The Centre for the Study of Social Work Practice, Columbia University School of Social Work	Ronald Feldman
	Hamovitch Center for Science in the Human Services, University of Southern California School of Social Work	Haluk Soydan
	Willma and Albert Musher Program	Ed Mullen

Notes

a Referred to as Intsoceval.

b Unless otherwise stipulated, information on these research centres is available at http://www.intsoceval.org/centres/index.asp

(SCIE) in the UK, Columbia University in the USA and the Institute for Evidence-based Practice (IMS)[12] in Sweden, which incorporates the Centre for Evaluation of Social Services (CUS) – these centres have not played a pivotal role in the evaluation of practice initiatives (see Cheetham *et al.* 1998) and, more recently, in the diffusion of evidence-based practice in their home countries. It seems then that Intsoceval is largely a church for the converted, a support group for those trying to spread the word of practice evaluation and evidence-based practice further afield. With the afore-mentioned exceptions, they do not generate 'gold standard' evidence via systematic reviews. This is largely the role of the C2 and SCIE, though IMS researchers work closely with C2. Thus, evidence-based practice has gained uneven acceptance in Europe, though Sweden and the UK are important nodes of diffusion, which might accelerate with the location of the Campbell Collaboration head office in Norway (known as the Nordic C2 or NC2). However, as we shall see from the case study of Norway below, most Norwegian social workers do not seem to be informed about developments in evidence-based policy and practice.

Netherlands

The debate on evidence-based practice has only just begun in the Netherlands (Garretsen *et al.* 2005). Advocates of evidence-based practice there link it solidly to intervention effectiveness and enhancement of the accountability of services delivered within the Dutch welfare sector, to match developments within health-care. From their perspective, evidence is built through practice evaluation. Despite the fact that various scholars have identified the lack of evidence of effectiveness within Dutch welfare practice, nevertheless, some managers, team leaders and social workers are supportive of evidence-based practice defined as results-oriented practice, which means making methods more measurable and using tested methods of effectiveness. However, there is resistance from welfare practitioners who argue that their work is not quantifiable and, furthermore, that it is hemmed in by legal and bureaucratic restraints. Skeptical managers worry that lack of proven effectiveness will lead to cuts in services. Most evaluations are internal and based on client feedback rather than formal objective research. Another problem is the changeability of the welfare sector, which makes it difficult for practitioners to benefit from proven experience or to make improvements based on past experience. Finally, practitioners lack research expertise or the ability to evaluate their practice systematically, not to mention the ability to locate or critically appraise research.

Nevertheless, there is an evolving network of organizations promoting evidence-based practice, such as the Dutch Scientific Centre for Transformation in Care and Welfare at the University of Tilburg; the Trimbos Institute, i.e., the Netherlands Institute for Mental Health and Addiction (NIMHA); the Addiction Research Institute; Netherlands Youth Institute; and the Vervey-Jonker Institute, from which Willem Melief has been a key contributor to Intsoceval. Also, the Netherlands has a strong Cochrane Centre. As in Australia, evidence-based practice is more likely to be implemented by practitioners closest to or within the health sector (Plath 2006). Most of these organizations have the following aims: to generate scientific knowledge in their area of practice; to monitor policy development and lobby policy-makers and politicians; to conduct research on the organization, accessibility, quality and effectiveness of services; to develop practice guidelines; to provide training; and to raise the awareness of the general population on knowledge related to their problem area. Henk Garretsen, whose main area of research is addictions, believes that, for the full benefits of evidence-based practice to be realized in the Netherlands, *partnerships between service developers and service users* are needed, as well as partnerships between researchers based in research institutes and universities, and practitioners in the welfare sector (Garretsen *et al.* 2005).

Sweden

A mixed picture of evidence-based practice in social work emerges from the literature on Sweden. Bergmark and Lundström (1998, 2000, 2002) found that social workers did not read the professional literature and were not interested in research. However, their more recent studies show that there has been some change with more positive attitudes towards research, welcoming its propensity to strengthen social work practice, and an increased number of social workers reporting that they have read professional literature, at least in the northwestern municipalities of Stockholm, the area they studied (Bergmark and Lundström 2007, 2008). With key social agency directors strongly supporting evidence-based practice, one wonders whether social workers are eager to give the appearance of moving with the times. Sundell *et al.* (2008) reported on a small study where seven of the ten agency directors interviewed expressed a keen interest in evidence-based interventions, which were used more frequently in child and adolescent services and substance abuse treatment units, while standardized assessment instruments were more common in units for older adults and for individuals with substance abuse problems. The most important factors driving the use of evidence-based interventions included recommendations from state agencies, such as the National Board of Health and Welfare, explicit directives from high-ranking decision-makers and an expressed interest among colleagues within organizations supportive of evidence-based practice. Certainly there are strong pressures toward evidence-based practice from government. For example, a commission established by the Swedish Ministry of Education recommended in its official report that evidence-based practice be compulsory professional practice. This recommendation entailed practitioners keeping up-to-date with professional literature and developing expertise in evidence-based practice: 'The organization of the social services must support the development of expertise within different fields. Platforms [supporting] … better collaboration between research and practice must be developed' (Statens Offentliga Utredningar (SOU) 2008: 83). Another recommendation was that research on outcomes, quality and effectiveness of social services 'should be specially supported for the next six years within a frame of a national program. Swedish Council for Working Life and Social Research (FAS) should be responsible for the implementation of the program' (SOU 2008: 111). The commission estimated that the program would cost 17 million SEK per annum for the ensuing six-year period and recommended that FAS be allocated a budget to enable it to fund experimental research and intervention studies in association with major national development projects. Clearly then, the Swedish government is championing service evaluation and creating a research-oriented culture within which evidence-based practice is likely to thrive in Sweden.

While most social work faculty either do not understand research or are resistant to evidence-based practice (yielding a similar picture to that of Germany, outlined below), Swedish academic Verner Denvall (2008) believes that with the ongoing academization of social work, i.e., with the growing importance of research-based practice, it is likely that alliances between social work practice agencies and universities and research organizations will increase in the future. Organizations like SCIE in the UK (see Chapter 5), NC2 and those involved in Intsoceval, including Sweden's IMS, are collectively working to promote program evaluation and evidence-based practice. Policy-makers and agency directors are becoming increasingly convinced, mainly through the work first of Haluk Soydan and now IMS's current director, Knut Sundell, under Soydan's guidance, that evidence-based practice should be widely adopted within the Swedish social services.

Finland

This same trend is evident in Finnish social work, which, though it favours post-modern perspectives and qualitative research (Rostila and Piirainen, in Thyer and Kazi 2004, see Karvinen 1996, 1999; Karvinen, Pösö and Satka 1999), and casts social work practice very much within the problem-solving mode. Thus where research is taught this is the methodology of choice with the result that quantitative research and evidence-based practice are greeted with a great deal of scepticism. In any event, there is little empirical work on which to draw and what there is relates more directly to service evaluation. Nevertheless, those working to promote evidence-based practice in Finland, such as Mikko Mantysaari at the University of Jyvaskyla, also construe it within a practice evaluation or 'what works' agenda. As stated by Rostila and Piirainen (in Thyer and Kazi 2004: 208), '(Re)constructing social work as problem-solving activity in co-operation with clients is a prerequisite for evaluating the outcomes of social work for its clients .... There is an urgent need to evaluate the outcomes of social work in practice settings'.

Despite such ambivalence about evidence-based practice, in some quarters efforts to bridge the gap between science and practice are proceeding apace. Two multi-site RCTs on multi-systemic therapy (MST), a treatment used for antisocial behaviour and conduct disorder in children and adolescents, were conducted in Norway and Sweden (Gustle *et al.* 2007, 2008; Ogden and Halliday-Boykins 2004; Ogden and Hagen 2006; Ogden *et al.* 2007, 2008).[13] Gustle *et al.* (2008: 111) reported on their study of the attitudes of community-based social workers and their supervisors towards the Swedish research project, as well as towards use of MST. They found that:

> ... a large majority of participants were positive toward the research project, felt sufficiently informed, and thought that the implementation occurred at an appropriate pace. Likewise, participants felt positively toward the adoption of MST as a treatment method, toward evidence-based research in general, and in their affinity toward community–family-based services.

However, they also found that 'social workers differed in their practice attitudes'. They attributed this to 'the influence of top-down implementation, differences in experience, and differences due to the position [they] held' (*ibid.*).

Norway

Most of the discussions and papers on evidence-based practice in the social work literature from Sweden, Finland, Norway and Denmark are in Scandinavian languages and are, therefore, published in domestic journals within each country. There has been some discourse on evidence-based practice in the social work literature over the last ten years. In the Nordic countries, most of these social work discussions have had an epistemological focus, being more concerned with new ways of understanding knowledge-making rather than embracing evidence-based practice. There is also a strong focus on the democratization of services that does not fit neatly with a strong scientific perspective or narrow understanding of evidence-based practice and 'gold standard' research. As Gambrill (2006b) has noted, the focus on intervention outcomes to minimize harm to clients is too narrow for social work where any harm, no matter how minimal, is unethical.

In keeping with this strong hermeneutical tradition, Marthinsen (2004) proposes an approach which combines reflexivity with the principles of the learning organization. He perceives an ideological struggle between the phenomenological approach, which supports communitarian ideas, and a scientific one set against a neo-liberal, atomistic new positivism. His focus, however, is the dependence of what he calls a 'mind for learning' and 'on a learning organization with certain qualities and tools that enable the organizational structure to extract knowledge from practice' (Marthinsen 2004: 54). A mind for learning is a 'mind for research' or 'research mindedness'. Such a mind seeks not to make practitioners 'slaves of science' but to create a space for knowledge-making in practice. He sees learning as a scaffolded process, with the highest level involving experience in the craft as well as skills in knowledge-production combined with a deep understanding of epistemology within the profession or discipline concerned, in this case social work. His goal is to understand 'how research as well as practice can respond to the growing interest in making services more scientific' (Marthinsen 2004: 57) while avoiding the political rhetoric which supports efficiency and cost-effectiveness and justifies service cuts. There is clearly resistance to and misunderstanding of the evidence-based practice approach, which is not just about keeping practitioners up-to-date with research or making them research minded, but relates more broadly to 'quality care and the minimisation of ... [clinical] error, the ethical and equitable provision of services, as well as the effective and efficient distribution of scarce resources from a public health perspective' (Leung 2001: 117).

It seems, however, from this literature, that social work practitioners are out of touch with developments in evidence-based policy in the fields of mental health, child welfare and education in Norway. Evidence-based policy is being promoted through the Centre for the Prevention and Treatment of Violence and Traumatic Stress, the Regional Centres for Child and Adolescent Mental Health, the Norwegian Knowledge Centre for the Health Services, and the Norwegian Centre for Child Behavioural Development (Ogden 2008). Within the health area, for example, research has influenced policy development, and enhanced awareness of evidence-based policy decisions in the development of interdisciplinary guidelines for clinicians working with children of mentally ill or drug-abusing parents, and prevalence studies in the area of mental health of children and youth have influenced political decisions and led to massive investment in research and development both at the national and regional levels. There are, however, large unmet needs in several areas of research, such that while political and policy decisions might sometimes be research informed, they hardly qualify for being research based. In education, a new initiative is being launched in which the Directorate of Education is establishing a division of implementation and change in order to improve the implementation and translation of research findings. The Ministry of Education is considering whether to establish a knowledge-producing organization (a clearinghouse or knowledge centre) or to strengthen already established research institutions in the field of educational research.

The implementation and evaluation of evidence-based programs in the treatment of children and youth with serious behaviour problems offers another example of how research is influencing policy and practice. In 1998 a governmental initiative was launched in Norway to strengthen services, practitioner competence and empirical research relating to children and young people with serious behavioural problems. Priority funding was given to the adoption and implementation of evidence-based family and community treatment programs in child welfare services, e.g., multi-systemic therapy (MST), parental management training (PMTO) and the school-wide support program (PALS). This work dates back to 1998, when a research unit, funded by the Ministry of Child and Family Affairs, was established at the Institute of Psychology, University of Oslo, to integrate research and practice so as to increase multi-disciplinary knowledge and promote clinical competence in the prevention and treatment of serious behaviour problems in children and young people. Consequently, a national implementation of US evidence-based programs was initiated and, in 2003, the Norwegian Centre for Child Behavioural Development, affiliated with the University of Oslo, was established with funding from the ministries and directorates of child welfare, mental health and education. The implementation of the child and youth (behavioural) development policy involved a combined top-down and bottom-up implementation strategy. A national centre was established to coordinate policy, practice and research. In the practice stream, therapists and practitioners were recruited through the regular service systems and a comprehensive therapist-practitioner training and supervision program was initiated. An extensive quality assurance system to monitor compliance, productivity and outcomes began, along with research on child and adolescent behavioural change and on the quality of program implementation in daily practice. One of the evidence-based treatment programs introduced into Norway's child welfare services was MST (see Ogden and Halliday-Boykins 2004; Ogden and Hagen 2006; Ogden *et al*. 2007, 2008). By 2006, 482 treatments had been initiated and evaluated. Among them, 86.5 per cent proved successful, 6.5 per cent resulted in

placement in out-of-home care and 7.1 per cent were unsuccessful, with participants dropping out of treatment. By 2007, there were twenty-three locally-based
teams implementing this program. By the same time, the extensive PMTO, which
was initiated in 1999, had trained and certified more than 200 therapists from all
health regions and approximately 1,500 families had undergone treatment. PALS,
modelled on the School-wide Positive Behavior Support (PBS) program developed
at the University of Oregon and used in combination with PMTO, aimed to
strengthen students' capacity for coping with developmental challenges at school.
Starting with an initial pilot of four schools, by 2007 it had been implemented in
ninety-one schools across Norway.

Norway thus provides an interesting example of evidence-based policy attempting to link research, policy and practice in high-priority problem areas. This has
involved long-term funding commitments at the political policy level for the
large-scale implementation of several evidence-based interventions, as described
above. The approach has been multi-pronged. There has been sustained support
from the program developers for the selected, empirically validated programs and
positive feedback from families, those involved in program delivery and the media.
Full-scale replication outcome studies are being conducted and programs are being
systematically monitored.

However, several challenges remain, among them the extent to which those
implementing the programs are staying true to their original form, which is an
important factor in valid and reliable outcome studies. Further, there is, as yet,
a lack of broad acceptance of evidence-based practice among policy-makers
and practitioners. Thus integrating an evidence-based practice approach in daily
practice remains a challenge.[14]

Germany

A similar skepticism to that identified by Marthinsen in Norway is evident in
German social work. Heinz Kindler (2008), from the German Youth Institute,
attributes this to three possible factors. The first is ideological and inheres in the
deep-rooted idealistic philosophical tradition in Germany, which still prevails in
schools of social work in the guise of phenomenological and critical theory. This
gives rise to a distrust of instrumental reason – and technical rationality – which
is strongly identified with evidence-based practice (see Otto and Ziegler 2008
below and Spratt and Houston 1999, which typify this Germanic approach). For the
most part, social work education, rather than preparing students for any particular
practice context, aims to empower professionals 'by helping them *understand* and
reflect upon important ideas, experiences, societal developments, and their clients'
position within [socio-political] processes' (Kindler 2008: 322 emphasis added).
Thus critical reflection – or reflexive practice – is an important social work ability
which can be done whether or not empirical research is available to practitioners.
In short, 'the time-consuming, cost-intensive, empirical study of narrow concrete
problems … is not valued' (*ibid.*).

Kindler's (2008) second explanation for German social work's resistance to evidence-based practice is pragmatic. Few German social work professors, despite their deep understanding of research epistemology and methodology, have ever done or published high-quality empirical research. Liel and Kindler (2006), in their study of 500 German social work publications over a five-year period, did not find a single systematic review. Two controlled studies were located, along with four explanatory studies. Most empirical studies were illustrative (n=46) or descriptive (n=39). In brief, 'Germany simply does not examine [the] effects of social work' (Kindler 2008: 322).

Kindler's (2008) third explanation is political. Practice evaluation, outcome measurement or evidence-based practice is simply not part of German federal legislation, though this is changing: 'The most recent federal document on the development of programs to prevent abuse and neglect during early childhood explicitly states that scientific research on the effects of early prevention should be conducted, and at least one randomized controlled trial has already started' (Kindler 2008: 322).

Kindler (2008), whose main area of research is child protection, an area where there is a growing international empirical literature, is a strong proponent of evidence-based practice. Based on a systematic review of this international literature, the German Youth Institute has published a *Handbook of child protection practice* (Kindler *et al.* 2006). As already mentioned, he notes the importance of *staying close to frontline workers* – many of whom in German child protection have social work qualifications – since it is they who use and validate the results of their research.

Otto and Ziegler (2008) present an entirely different view, questioning whether evidence-based practice is right for social work or, more specifically, whether the 'Campbell-style' research it advocates suits the problems and issues with which social workers deal. In 2006, the Centre for Social Service Studies of the University of Bielefeld, where Hans-Uwe Otto is the director, hosted an international conference to debate this issue. They see the thrust to evidence-based practice as running too close for comfort to the goals of new public management, though they accept that it is unfair to blame evidence-based social work for the 'technocratic managerial developments in the organization of social work' (Otto and Ziegler 2008: 274). They acknowledge that proponents of evidence-based practice are opposed to managerialism but, nonetheless, point out that 'It would be naïve to ignore the similarities between evidence-based protocols, actuarial calculations, and the *regulating* tools that represent some of the cornerstones of managerial bureaucratization' (*ibid.*, emphasis added). Indeed evidence-based social work is likely to benefit from the 'managerial quest to make social work "auditable"' since it has 'contributed to the new belief that methodologically rigorous impact evaluations are not an unaffordable luxury, but a necessary investment for *governing* social work practice to enhance its efficiency' (Otto and Ziegler 2008: 274, emphasis added). Otto and Ziegler (2008: 276) note that, for the full benefits of empirically validated practice to be felt, evidence-based social work has to be *standardized*. However, evidence-based practice, as its definition articulates, combines standardized evidence with practitioner skill and client values, creating leeway for flexibility in the application of evidence. Hence Otto and Ziegler's (2008: 276) conclusion about 'cookbook' social work and its threat to professional reflexivity and autonomy must be regarded with caution. As we saw in Kindler's (2008) evaluation of German social work above, professional reflexivity is highly valued but the 'dissemination of evidence-based guidelines' need not mean the erosion of 'reflexive professionalism in social work'. Recent conferences have probed these issues, which are important in the implementation of evidence-based practice.[15]

Asia–Pacific region

A different picture of receptivity to evidence-based practice is discernible in the Asia–Pacific region. Leung (2001), though he is writing about evidence-based medicine, provides a clue to the way in which evidence-based practice in other fields is likely to be embraced in Hong Kong and mainland China and, perhaps, in the Asia–Pacific region generally. There evidence-based medicine and evidence-based practice in related health fields – like nursing (Yin King Lee 2003), occupational therapy (Dasari 2003) and psychology (especially in relation to cognitive behaviour therapy – see below) – are gaining momentum, with evidence-based practice now part of educational curricula in Hong Kong. Evidence-based practice is promoted by Hong Kong's Hospital Authority, and has been since 1998. In 2000, it became institutionalized with the establishment of the Clinical Effectiveness Unit. The Hong Kong Hospital Authority has run training and professional development workshops and programs conducted by overseas experts.

Speaking of which, in 2008, Haluk Soydan and Dan Hester from the University of Southern California organized the first international conference on evidence-based practice and policy-making – defined as practice based on scientific research findings to make better and more informed decisions that affect people's lives – for the social sciences in Beijing in collaboration with Peking University's Institute of Population Research. The two-day conference, held over 17–18 March, was attended by more than 100 Chinese scholars and government officials. This was the first step of providing a framework for the establishment of a Chinese Centre on Evidence-based Practice in the Social Sciences at Peking University, which would be the first of its kind in Asia. The centre would enable Chinese and US researchers to collaborate effectively, using internationally recognized approaches to scientific documentation. It would also contribute significantly to joint research and the ability of social scientists to have an impact on policy-making and professional interventions on vital social policy issues that affect the well-being of citizens in both countries. The importance of access to information on 'what works' was emphasized, as it allowed practitioners to select treatments that would most likely be helpful and least likely be harmful. This was more desirable in the human services than relying solely on rules, single observations or helping traditions. The ideology of evidence-based practice is, thus, becoming a major driving force impacting upon clinical practice education, policy-making and scientific research. Chinese people are intensely interested in what generates and constitutes high-quality scientific evidence. To this end, the workshop provided information on evidence-based practice methodology. Haluk Soydan from the USC School of Social Work, Robert Boruch from the University of Pennsylvania Graduate School of Education, and Youping Li, the director of the Chinese Cochrane Centre in Chengdu, China, led workshops on 'clearinghouses' around the world which compile, assess and disseminate reliable information in specific fields, such as social work and education. The workshops also examined the way in which systematic research reviews were produced and how they might be adopted for use in China. Soydan talked about the Campbell Collaboration:

> ... an organization [which] he co-founded that brings together international scholars who contribute to making reliable research information available and accessible to policymakers, practitioners and the public. The researchers conduct rigorous systematic reviews of research to make sense of large, fragmented and sometimes conflicting knowledge in an effort to identify what works and what does not. The organization's eventual goal is to build a comprehensive database that will enable people who are reviewing the effectiveness of interventions to weigh a thorough body of evidence. Soydan believes that optimistic Chinese social scientists will embrace the idea of translating evidence into their clinical practice and policymaking based on the experiences of the Chinese Cochrane Center, a sister organization dedicated to evidence-based health care. 'I am personally dedicated to this endeavor and eager to see it move forward,' Soydan said. 'We begin meeting with Peking University this summer about how to develop a feasible infrastructure in China that will support interdisciplinary projects from all areas of the university and across multiple professions' (http://www.usc.edu/uscnews/stories/15096.html).

It is likely that the evidence-based practice will grow quite quickly in mainland China, given that Hong Kong already has a well-established evidence-based practice infrastructure, including a comprehensive web-based electronic gateway (eKG) (Leung 2001). Furthermore, in China there are cultural precedents which go back to 'the reign of Chinese Emperor Qianlong (1736–1799) in the Qing Dynasty where the method of *kaozheng xue* ("practising evidentiary research") was used to dispel dogmatic traditional teachings and to reinterpret ancient Confucian texts based on documented facts' (Leung 2001: 116).

Leung (2001) believes that practice has yet to catch up with the rapid technological advances that have catapulted evidence-based practice to international attention. He cites figures which show that the time lag between research and its application to practice is fifteen to twenty years (see also the results of the NIMH (2000) reported in Brekke *et al.* 2007 and Soydan 2007). He sees evidence-based practice as being especially relevant in Asia, where there is a huge demand for services and where ways need to be found to assist people requiring urgent attention but who are instead getting trapped in long medical centre queues. Evidence-based practice offers a way 'to make better informed decisions, thereby maximizing the health impact of every scarce dollar' (Leung 2001: 117).

One gets the sense when reading these few sources on evidence-based practice in China that the diffusion theorists are correct and the uptake of evidence-based practice in this region is only a matter of time. Chinese policy-makers are eager to base policy on research and it is likely that this will greatly influence the development of social work practice in China which, to date, involves nearly 200 social work education programs with no formal jobs for graduates (Gray 2005, 2008).

Similar trends are evident in the Asia–Pacific more broadly, with the establishment of the Asia Pacific Center for Evidence-Based Medicine based in Manila in the Philippines.[16] The Center holds conferences and workshops on matters relating to evidence-based practice. The seventh Asia Pacific Evidence-Based Medicine and Nursing Workshop and Conference was held in Singapore in January 2009.

Martis *et al.* (2008), in their survey of knowledge and perception on the access to evidence-based practice and clinical practice change among maternal and infant health practitioners (n=660) in South East Asia, reported on the information technology (IT) constraints facing practitioners, i.e., nurses and midwives. Less than half had ease of access to IT; over 20 per cent had no access at all and more than 50 per cent had never used IT health information. Just less than half had heard of the Cochrane Library and of these, 51 per cent had access but the majority did not use it or used it less than once a month. While 58 per cent had heard of evidence-based practice, the majority did not understand the concept. The most frequent sites accessed were Google and PubMed. Only 27 per cent had heard of the WHO Reproductive Health Library. Nevertheless, most expressed willingness to participate in professional development workshops on evidence-based practice.

In Japan, a few US- or UK-trained academics – such as Keiji Akiyama, Dean of the College of Humanities at Kanto Gakuin University in Yokohama and Matsujiro Shibano, Professor of the School of Sociology at Kwansei Gakuin University in Tokyo – have been instrumental in initiating evidence-based social work in Japan. Its adoption, however, is severely hampered by language difficulties as it has not yet been translated into the Japanese social work literature, though some Japanese writers have published internationally (Akiyama and Buchanan 2007; Shibano 2004, 2007[17]) and there is some collaboration with the EPPI Centre at the University of London (see http://eppi.ioe.ac.uk/cms/).

In Australasia – Australia and New Zealand – evidence-based practice is most advanced in relation to medicine and allied health professions (Gale 1998), even though some practitioners remain cautious about this approach (Leach 2006). In Australia, the National Institute for Clinical Studies based in Melbourne develops clinical guidelines and protocols to assist clinicians in applying the latest evidence, and in New Zealand, the New Zealand Guidelines Group (NZGG), established in 1996 by the National Health Committee (NHC), is an informal network of expertise and information on guidelines development and implementation. In 1999, the NZGG became an independent incorporated society with its main office in Wellington and a satellite office in Auckland.

There has been progress, too, in psychology. In 2006, the First Asian Cognitive Behaviour Therapy (CBT) Conference was held as a joint venture between the schools of psychology at Queensland University and the Chinese Hong Kong University, the theme of which was evidence-based assessment, theory and treatment. The conference sought to examine evidence-based assessment and theory – noting the over-emphasis on the efficacy of treatment – and to examine ways of researching CBT on Asian samples, given that this mode of intervention was widely used in Asian countries.

The second conference held in October 2008 in Bangkok, addressed the cross-cultural integration in CBT, moving across the boundaries. Its program notes that while CBT has been widely accepted and used by mental health professionals in the Western world, where the effectiveness of the therapy has been shown empirically and is beyond question, and increasingly in Asia, practitioners report that cultural differences between the Eastern and Western worlds interfere with the effectiveness of CBT. Hence there is a need to examine cultural issues relating to the use of CBT in non-Western contexts.

Similar claims might be made about evidence-based practice in indigenous contexts, especially when it fails to take account of indigenous and local knowledges or of research methodologies consistent with indigenous worldviews or local cultures (Denzin *et al.* 2008; Gray *et al.* 2008; Fejo-King 2005; Smith 1999). At this stage, evidence-based practice necessarily involves Western models of practice and most literature on the subject emanates from English-speaking countries where professionals are likely to practise and teach in this way. As we have seen, this creates difficulties for countries not conversant with English in accessing the evidence-based practice literature and databases, such as those kept by C2 and SCIE.

Within Australasian university research environments, there are strong external pressures on academics to engage far more actively in research and to generate research income. This does not necessarily translate into evidence-based practice, however, especially within social work, where it has been greeted with considerable suspicion by social work academics and practitioners alike, who are strongly motivated by social justice values and a critical ideology. Yet the language of evidence has become commonplace within human services in Australia and, as Plath (2006) notes, in Australian social work evidence-based practice is most likely to be found where social work is practised within health and mental health contexts. Nevertheless, social work in Australia has been influenced by the literature on and debates about evidence-based practice originating in the USA and the UK. Similar to other countries, divisions and debates have occurred within the profession that reflect the tensions between experimental and interpretative research-based knowledge for practice (Gray and McDonald 2006; Plath 2006; Scott 2002).

Within social work education, there is an emphasis on the critical appraisal of research to inform practice, but schools of social work have not adopted evidence-based practice as a fundamental principle for social work education. The Australian Association of Social Workers (AASW) initiated an evidence-based practice subgroup, but this has had little impact on social work practice and Australian social workers are often unclear about the implications of evidence-based practice for how social work is practised (Murphy and McDonald 2004). The language of evidence has, however, been embraced at a government policy level, where programs and policy initiatives are often couched in terms of being 'evidence-based'. Human service organizations receiving government funding grants are required to justify their services in terms of evidence that demonstrates effective outcomes. Despite this, Australia does not have the research infrastructure to produce extensive local research findings or a research database to support such requirements. Human service providers make use of international databases from the UK and USA to identify relevant research to inform practice. This generally entails interpreting transferability to the particular social and organizational features of Australian service provision. Human service providers also draw upon available local research, which often comprises internal, practice-based evaluations conducted in particular organizations. In order to maintain funding there is an expectation that evidence for effectiveness is provided, but there is no rigour in establishing the nature or extent of that evidence. There is currently much rhetoric about evidence but, in practice, this often equates to a situation where any evidence will suffice.

Other international contexts

Israel

In Israel, Ronen (in Thyer and Kazi 2004) reports that social workers continue to ignore what little evidence there is on EBIs, preferring to practise from a normative or value-based stance (Rosen 1994). Also, what research exists – mostly in the health, mental health and military fields – is not based on experimental comparison groups or single system designs. Such studies are rare in social work (Auslander 2000). This is unlikely to change in the near future, given that there is very little uptake of research by postgraduate – Masters – students, mainly because of the social work curriculum, university faculty, field supervisors, the structure, role and aims of social work schools, and so on, none of which has systematically embraced evidence-based practice. Overall, social work is aimed at practice not research. Hence there is a lack of resources, training and knowledge for evidence-based practice. Those engaged in research prefer intervention research models which identify a problem, design and implement an intervention and evaluate it through use of single-case designs and controlled outcome studies. Some advances have been made in studying the relationship between behaviour problems and self-control mechanisms in children (Ronen 1994). Another group of researchers, Benbenishty and colleagues (in Ronen, in Thyer and Kazi 2004), believe that instruments to assess outcome should be designed in collaboration with clients and the practitioners who will use them. They have developed an 'integrated information system' which follows an action learning model wherein services are monitored, results are shared and learning ensues from experience. For the most part, however, Israeli social work practice is not evidence-based and is unlikely to be in the near future.

Canada

Writing from Canada, Holosko (in Thyer and Kazi 2004) reports that Canadian schools of social work, by and large, do not – and have not – promoted evidence-based practice, despite developments in medicine led by the McMaster Group. Nor does evidence-based practice shape social work practice, despite Holosko's own research on music intervention with alcoholics. In short, empirically based, let alone evidence-based, practice in Canada is virtually non-existent and this is unlikely to change. However, the work of Jim Barber at the University of Toronto and that of Aron Shlonsky and colleagues following Barber's return to Australia, show promising developments in evidence-based practice in Canada. The minutes of the Campbell Collaboration on social work in Canada[18] report that the Steering Group:

> ... voted to approve two proposals for two new C2 partner organizations: University of Toronto School of Social Work (Aron Shlonsky, lead) and York University in Toronto (David Phipps, lead). A third proposal for a C2 partner organization will be voted by 30 June 2007; this proposal is from the Canadian group CanKnow (Phil Abrami, lead) and its leaders have been active in C2 and the C2 Education group. The SG will initiate discussions with the partner organizations in order to specify more clearly what each partner can expect to contribute to and receive from C2.

Some commonalities across contexts

1 Evidence-based practice does not exist in practice, and consistent studies across international contexts show that social workers neither do nor use research.
2 Evidence-based practice as an idea is strongest the more aligned social work is to the health and mental health sectors.
3 There is a growing network of research organizations working to promote evidence-based practice in social work.
4 Most research being conducted relates to the evaluation of country-based public services at various levels of delivery or to particular problem areas, such as addictions, especially alcoholism, immigration and refugees (e.g., Denmark) and family violence.
5 There is a growing focus on the generation of evidence but little attention being paid to end users.

Global mobilization of evidence-based practice

As outlined at the outset, actor network theory provides valuable insights into the local–global actor networks that surround evidence-based practice. The mobilization, interaction and disintegration of the evidence-based practice network can be understood in relation to network actor 'power to' change the practice of social work internationally through the exercise of leadership in the process of network formation and maintenance. We have seen how key actors – individuals and organizations – repeatedly appear in discussions of evidence-based practice in various countries. Actor network theory offers a dynamic, positive, enactive understanding of power as a micro practice – not the static conception of 'power over' others but the 'power to' effect innovation and change within a dynamic network. It offers explicit understanding of the political interactions of multiple stakeholders, of collective 'politicking' through a *global network* 'that is built up, deliberately or otherwise, and that generates a space, a period of time, and a set of resources' (Callon and Law 1982: 22), which can be seen as external to the project, the project being evidence-based practice conducted by practitioners at the coalface. The *local network* is the internal set of relations necessary to the successful production and implementation of an innovation, which, in this case is evidence-based practice. So what we are interested in with regard to the local network is the relation of the actors *inside* the evidence-based practice project, the educators who teach it and the practitioners who implement it. In terms of Callon and Law's (1982: 46) global–local framework, the success or failure of a project hinges on three interrelated factors:

1   The capacity of the project to build and maintain a global network that will for a time provide resources of various kinds in the expectation of an ultimate return.
2   The ability of the project to build a local network using the resources provided by the global network to ultimately offer a material, economic, cultural or symbolic return to actors lodged in the global network.
3   The capacity of the project to impose itself as an obligatory point of passage between the two networks.

The 'obligatory point of passage' is a single locus that controls the transactions between global and local networks and the flow of objects or intermediaries, such as documents and physical artefacts, between them. What ensues, then, is a global set of resource providers and a local set of implementers. Within evidence-based practice, the C2s are the 'global' actors and could play a far more influential role in attaching local actors to global networks. By the same token, local actors need to more energetically mobilize local actor networks to adopt evidence-based practice. As outlined previously, this entails active engagement with practitioners and a bringing together of all local actors into a consolidated local network interacting with the global C2s.

From the case studies presented above, based on Callon and Law's (1982) framework presented in Figure 4.1, one would have to be extremely skeptical about the strength of the evidence-based practice project which lacks a solid global network – an obligatory point of passage – and has a minimal degree of mobilization in local networks, i.e., those within particular countries. As we shall see with the case study which follows in Chapter 5, a strong national network like SCIE has the propensity to mobilize and engage local actors but such a strong coordinating body is lacking in the USA and elsewhere. There are too many organizations representing diverse

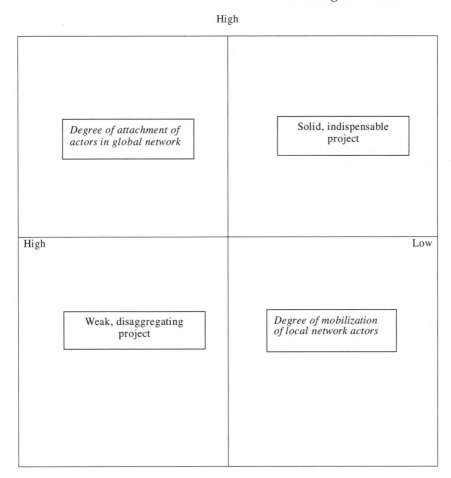

High

Degree of attachment of
actors in global network

Solid, indispensable
project

High   Low

Weak, disaggregating
project

Degree of mobilization
of local network actors

Low

Figure 4.1 Mobilization of local and global networks.

Source: Callon and Law (1982).

interest groups in the USA and only a loose network of research bodies connected through Intsoceval in Europe. One might conclude, then, that it is early days for the global and local evidence-based practice project.

Conclusion

In conclusion, this chapter focused on the diffusion or dispersal of evidence-based social work within a global context. It showed that the recent history of evidence-based social work, which in its most accurate definition only enters social work at the turn of the century, while uneven and non-linear, is, in fact, part of the history of (technological) resources and innovations scattered along networks to accelerate the mobility, adherence and cohesion of mappings that make possibile the standardization of social work interventions. But there is a long way to go.

Through a process of drift, diffusion and dispersion, evidence-based social work aims to persuade educators and practitioners to appreciate the importance of scientific alternatives. Ultimately, for it to really take hold, a much more coordinated approach would have to be taken to make interventions standard across time and place and to create a durable and mobile set of protocols that would guide decision-making when combined with infrastructural resources. The adaptation system which evidence-based social work depends upon may be seen as a vehicle of dispersal and diffusion which transforms specific developments in local contexts into global ones. We demonstrated that the diffusion of evidence-based social work across an international context is best understood in asymmetrical terms, with the evidence-based practice innovation originating exclusively in 'progressive' centres (the USA and UK, see Chapter 5) from which it spreads. Diffusion theory holds that the pattern of adoption resembles a bell-shaped curve beginning with a small percentage of innovators (2.5 per cent) to early adopters (13.5 per cent) and so on to early and late majorities of 34 per cent, coming down again with the laggards at 16 per cent. Over time, however, the pattern of diffusion resembles an S-shaped curve beginning with a period of slow, gradual growth followed by a period of dramatic growth before levelling out again.

We have seen how the diffusion of evidence-based social work is dependent first on risk-taking innovators, followed by the articulation of 'receptors' – an organizational infrastructure comprising institutions, policies and practices – which promote the innovation and are capable of generating standard applications. For instance, with Sweden and the Netherlands we saw that less emphasis is placed on the absorption of research for practice than on the actual process through which an evidence-based infrastructure is required to develop, step by step. In the USA we noted the emphasis on advocating for and teaching evidence-based practice. But missing from this, though recognized in some quarters, is the importance of the end user, i.e., the frontline practitioner, the subject of Chapter 7. However, first we examine the uptake of evidence-based practice in the UK in Chapter 5 and implementation in Chapter 6.

Notes

1 For example, in 2002 CSWE included evidence-based practice in its revised accreditation standards (EPAS, 2001, in Thyer 2004: 32). There is now a revised 2008 version.
2 http://www.cachildwelfareclearinghouse.org
3 In nomothetic research, the goal is to determine general laws and principles that apply to a population in general. A nomothetic research strategy samples systematically from the population and combines results across individuals. Its opposite is ideographic research, e.g., the case study method, which seeks to *understand* the individual. Its emphasis is the uniqueness of the individual rather than finding general laws.
4 These are freely available at http://www.apa.org/divisions/div12/journals.html#ESTs

5 http://www.ebbp.org

6 http://ebbp.org/syllabus.php

7 http://www.ebbp.org/competencies.html

8 http://www.socialworkers.org/advocacy/answer/default.asp

9 5th International Conference on Evaluation for Practice, Huddersfield, England, 2005; the 4th International Conference on Evaluation for Practice was held in Tampere, Finland, in 2002.

10 See NASW link to http://www.socialworkers.org/advocacy/answer/legislation/research.asp

11 Website maintained by SCIE – not updated since 2006 (http://www.intsoceval.org/)

12 http://www.sos.se/socialtj/cus/cuse/imse.htm

13 Asscher *et al.* (2007) have examined MST in criminal justice settings in the Netherlands. For a thorough review of research on MST, see Julia Littell (in Lindsey and Shlonsky 2008).

14 We are extremely grateful to Terje Ogden from the Norwegian Center for Child Behavioral Development, Unirand, University of Oslo, for this information and to Haluk Soydan for bringing this to our attention.

15 Translational research is now studying the implementation of evidence-based practice. This was the topic of a conference held in Stockholm – Conference on Implementation and Translational Research – on 16 October 2007. Conference papers are available at http://www.socialstyrelsen.se/IMS/implementeringskonferens.htm. The proceedings will be published in a special issue of *Research on Social Work Practice* in the summer of 2009 with Haluk Soydan as guest editor.

16 See http://www.apebm.com/

17 See also http://asr.kgu-jp.com/F1.php?F=F2&M=B1-7

18 http://camp.ostfold.net/artman2/uploads/1/Minutes_London_May2007.pdf

5   Forming the evidence network

How does evidence-based social work happen? This chapter further develops the diffusion analysis of Chapter 4. It provides some detailed observations on evidence-based social work in the UK through the lens of actor network theory. We use the UK case example to describe how diffusion occurs within a specific context by focusing on authorities of delimitation. These authorities comprise the social work research and policy and professional community, i.e., a network of institutions which possess their own rules. As a group of agencies and individuals, they constitute the social work profession – a sphere of activity with its own body of knowledge and standards of practice. These authorities are recognized by public opinion, the law, and government, and have become the major vehicle that named, designated, mobilized and formalized evidence as an object. We focus on organizations like the Social Care Institute of Excellence (SCIE), the Campbell Collaboration (C2) and the Centre for Evidence-Based Social Services (CEBSS) to undertake the actor network analysis of evidence-based networks in UK social work.

This chapter shows how the emergence of evidence-based social work in the UK is best conceived as a process of formalization whereby systems development and networks are central in legitimating the research program. We demonstrate how these complex processes can be conceptualized using actor network theory. By identifying various temporal markers and actors in the UK case study, we illustrate the way in which the evidence-based program is adapted, diffused and implemented.[1] It seems likely that the development of evidence-based social work is not based on traditional notions of innovation, as a process where clearly identified origins and trajectories are progressively mapped in some sequential order. Rather, it accumulates as a sort of 'situated drift' that is partly determined by the localness of the situation. Tracing the emergence of evidence-based social work in this way links to one of the fundamental claims in this book: that the research-to-practice program is not simply about how social workers use evidence to inform everyday decisions about interventions, but crucially about establishing formal systems and strategies of implementation. These form part of a panacea that authorizes and regulates the types of practice intervention that are permissible and those which are not.

Bruno Latour (1999) once claimed that it is not the Boeing 747 that flies us but the airline itself, with its entire ensemble of aligned human and non-human systems. Similarly, we contend that it is not a simple case of the evidence-based practitioner making the decision but rather the decision is the net effect of the articulation of evidence-based networks. Purposeful action becomes the property of institutions, systems and networks and not of objects or humans. We need to understand how evidence-based practice (EBP) is adopted, how it moves and how it progressively spreads to be transformed to an anticipated end point. Thus we shall see how an evidence-based intervention is the decision act that is linked together by a complex set of background influencing factors that are derived from a networked evidence system. In analyzing complex formalization pathways, evidence-based social work is thus best characterized as a socio-technical network or an emergent actor network. We discuss this aspect in more detail in Chapter 6 on processes of implementation, where we situate this evidence-based network as part of a wider trend based on the re-emergence of 'scientifically based research'. For now, however, we shall show how the development of evidence-based initiatives is framed, translated and mobilized by heterogeneous actor networks.

There is a need for more intensive micro studies of methodological and policy change associated with the evidence-based agenda, moving from global analysis to highly detailed and nuanced accounts of change as emergent networks. Such studies would allow us to understand how processes of improvization, purification and channelling are translated into local and national contexts, giving insights into the embedding of evidence-based methodology in day-to-day activities. It is shown that, at the core of the development of the evidence-based program, there are three strategies for innovation: how to enrol actors, how to control their behaviour and how to translate a normative agenda to fit the current circumstances. If we are to understand how these complex processes of iteration occur in the formalization of evidence-based practice in social work, and the way in which frontline interventions are narrowly framed as the end point of the process, then we need to know how the actor network gets put in place. Unlike other analyses on the emergence of evidence-based practice that focus on the methodology itself as a static entity that is adopted or not, our focus here is shifted to the emergent networks that surround the formalization process and the attempts by powerful stakeholders to enrol others by promoting it as a panacea for good professional practice in social work.

Adopting the talk?

We contend that the emergent evidence-based methodology does not just describe the realities of research, policy and interventions but is also involved in creating them. One author recalls an early winter morning induction session for a group of post-qualifying social workers to the local child care program they were due to start in the autumn of 2001. The convenor of the session was keen to convey the rigour and high degree of development of the program. During the fifteen-minute introductory talk, she uttered the term 'evidence' over fifty times. Specific usages included: 'best evidence', 'evidence for practice', 'using the evidence', 'only evidence counts', 'checking the evidence', 'empirical evidence', 'supporting decisions with evidence', 'making the evidence work', 'evidencing', 'evidentiary' and even 'the evidence from the evidence'. Putting aside the persuasive professional social-ization process at play in this example, the date roughly signifies the onset of the formalization of evidence-based practice in social work. It was also the date that *The New York Times Magazine* 'Year in Review' included evidence-based medi-cine as one of the most influential ideas of 2001.

The concept of formalization is a difficult one to grasp. In very simple terms it is about how a scientific innovation gets from point A to point Z as part of a formal process. An easy way to picture formalization is to think about the way in which eggs coagulate to bind ingredients when baking. It is a process whereby the protein of egg white, when heated, produces a clotting or thickening. A richer image is to think about a knotted ball of string or a tangled skein and the way in which the thread is woven. Untangling the knots is no easy task. However, once untangled the string is freed loose so that it can be dedicated to a particular task. The thread of knots may be contrasted with the pure, unknotted thread or the straight strands of the material. This image is helpful in thinking about ways in which innovative science becomes formalized as part of an iterative process of translation. It is also useful in considering how evidence-based practice in social work gradually comes to occupy a prominent place in considerations of what might constitute best practice. In simple terms, knot removing and untangling is crucial for the translation pathways of evidence-based practice. As we shall see, this is how we reach a stage where it becomes meaningful to talk about the implementation of evidence-based practice in social work. Implementation attempts in evidence-based practice are very revealing, because they demonstrate the formidable mobilization efforts that will have been incurred to diffuse the methodology. Moreover, as we shall see in Chapter 7, by the time evidence-based practice gets to the implementation stage, the formalization process will have travelled through various obligatory passage points, including institutions, policy and practice dimensions. With our analysis, it quickly becomes apparent that knowledge translation is much more than a straightforward process of taking evidence from research and applying it in frontline social work practice. In the sections below, we map some of the passages that evidence-based social work had to traverse to arrive at its current networked status.

UK case study: from knowledge to production

This section focuses on the UK case study, using actor network analysis. In par-ticular, it concentrates on how networked actors enrol other actors – humans or machines – through translations, i.e., by aligning their interests through arguments, negotiations, detours, or becoming indispensable.[2] We show how certain convergences and connections occur that allow the evidence network to acquire power through the number, extensiveness and stability of the connections routed through them. Powerful positions are defined during 'negotiations' and are created when certain actors enlist texts, artefacts and processes as 'enrolled' or 'allied' players and, in this the way, actors are obliged to remain faithful to their alliances (Callon 1991; Risan 1997). In doing so, the section demonstrates how the evidence-based actor network is formally established as a process that involves mobilization and translation through various pathways across the research, policy and intervention interface.

Where can we locate the origins of evidence-based social work in policy initiatives? In the UK, a concentrated focus on developing evidence-based social work followed the 1994 publication by the Department of Health Independent Review Group's influential *A wider strategy for research and development relating to the personal social services*. This report emphasized the need to promote a research culture at all levels, specifically to lay a basis for academic–practitioner partnerships, but focused particularly on weak links between research and practice interventions in social work. It was premised on the narrow management logic that surrounds evidence-based practice, whereby there are good and not-so-good ways to provide interventions in social services. If the good ways can be identified, systematized and consistently delivered to service users, then intervention outcomes will be optimized and costly inefficiency can be reduced or eliminated.

Translation of an innovation from one location to the next is not only about policy formation and implementation. It often involves key knowledge-broker actors or champions of a particular innovation. One of the most persistent and outspoken supporters of evidence-based practice in the UK over the past decade has been Geraldine Macdonald, who has had a close involvement with the Cochrane Collaboration (see next section) since the mid-1990s. One of the basic rules of actor network theory is 'to follow the actor' in defining the network. Latour (1996) likens this to a murder mystery novel in which questions are asked of each of the actors, and any subsequent directions and leads that may emerge from these initial questions are followed up by the detective. Indeed, as a rough guide to evaluating the changing fortunes of the evidence network in social work, one could do far worse than simply plotting this against Macdonald's shifting affiliations across the timeline. She is one of the central and most influential characters in the way in which the network unravels in the UK. While Macdonald was working at the University of Oxford, she served as the Archie Cochrane Research Fellow at Green College. Following this, at Bristol and subsequently Queens College Belfast, Macdonald held the powerful position of coordinating editor of the Cochrane Developmental, Psychosocial and Learning Problems Review Group established in 1998. What conception of evidence-based social work was Macdonald pursuing? In a slight modification of Sackett *et al.*'s definition of evidence-based medicine, Sheldon and Macdonald (1999: 4) claim that 'Evidence-based social care is the conscientious, explicit and judicious use of current best evidence in making decisions regarding the welfare of those in need of social services'. In her 1999 article, 'Evidence-based social care: wheels off the runway?', Macdonald (1999: 25) threw down the gauntlet by asserting that with British social services departments:

> Political ideology continues to play a major role in shaping policy and practice, despite a change of government. Sheltering beneath the ideological umbrella are more considered views of the need to rethink structures developed as a means of solving social problems and delivering service.

Implicit here was that, unless practitioners embraced the new evidence-based agenda, their professional identity would be challenged. Macdonald has repeatedly made the allegation that British social work is ideologically fused and politically contaminated. Unfortunately, we have not been able to find a definition of what she means by 'ideology', and we wonder if she might reflect on whether her own stance is ideologically driven.

As we shall see, Macdonald's contribution to the evidence-based agenda is revealing in helping us to plot the uneven trajectory of core elements of research for practice in social work. Her interest in evaluating the effects of social interventions rests on a particular appreciation of what constitutes social reality. She assumes that social reality is measurable, complacent and lends itself to statistical prediction. Macdonald is compelled by the prospects of evidence-based decision-making grounded on behaviourist principles of 'what works'.[3] Her slant on social work research has always been narrowly framed within a psychologistic perspective, from her early publication with Barbara Hudson, *Behavioural social work* (1986), to her later *Effective interventions for child abuse and neglect: an evidence-based approach to planning and evaluating interventions* (2001). In 1992 she published (with Sheldon) 'Contemporary studies of the effectiveness of social work', which used ninety-five experimental, quasi-experimental and pre-experimental studies, and in 1994 'Developing empirically-based practice in probation', both in the *British Journal of Social Work*. She later published two titles on 'what works' in relation to child protection and early years child development and, in a chapter called 'Social work and its evaluation: a methodological dilemma?' (1999b), she argued for the merits of randomized controlled trials (RCTs) for social work research. In her chapter 'Intervening with neglect' (2004), Macdonald insists that only certain kinds of evidence are acceptable. These include systematic reviews, RCTs and two-group studies. In line with this, Macdonald is sold on the idea of 'outcome research' informing frontline decisions.

There is a significant blind spot in Macdonald's approach to social research that rests on her adherence to a particular philosophy of science. Her approach is the descendant of a classical experimentalism that elevates quantitative-experimental methods to the top of the evidence-based hierarchy (see Figure 1.2), constraining other methods to a largely auxiliary role in the pursuit of a technocratic aim of achieving control, regulation and accumulating knowledge of 'what works'. In touting 'randomization' as the magic bullet to solve all problems, she completely ignores problems of establishing external validity for these studies, especially inconsistencies in implementing interventions across contexts and restricting the sample population and treatment to achieve the desired results (see Chapter 2). More on this below, but for now it is worth noting that there are significant problems with RCTs, not least that they are unable to establish the causal inference in social research they claim to achieve (see Briggs 2004; Korn 2006). Macdonald never questions the epistemological status for the brand of positivism she promotes, or acknowledges that it may be problematic. Nor does she consider whether the designs of effectiveness and evidence-based studies are intrinsically saturated with ambiguity, indeterminacy and contingency and the resulting 'truth claims' are necessarily 'constructions' and interpretations. More widely, Macdonald fails to consider whether the epistemological, ontological and methodological assumptions considered appropriate for clinical medicine may be inappropriate for non-biomedical health and social work. As a matter of validation, she never asks 'How do I know I'm right?' in critical epistemological terms. We return to this blind spot further on, especially in Chapter 6, where we examine the re-emergent scientism intrinsic to evidence-based agendas as a backlash against diverse forms of research and a feature of risk-avoidance culture in the wake of the 11 September 2001 terrorist attacks. For now, it will suffice to note that Macdonald's methodological conservativism is tagged to powerful gate-keeping processes and, as we show, is plugged directly into the emerging evidence network across a number of institutional affiliations and agenda-setting contexts.

The Campbell Collaboration

The formalization of the evidence-based agenda for medicine (EBM) in the UK began before developments in social work. However, as we have seen in Chapter 2, the term 'evidence-based medicine' is relatively new. It was researchers from McMaster University in Canada who began using the term during the 1990s. EBM was defined as 'a systemic approach to analyze published research as the basis of clinical decision making'.[4] The term was more formally defined by Sackett *et al.* in 1996 who stated that EBM was 'the conscientious and judicious use of current best evidence from clinical care research in the management of individual patients'. In the UK, the growth of EBM occurred against a backdrop of healthcare reform, managed care, performance culture, cost containment and quality improvement.

By far the most important development in mobilizing the EBM agenda and its networking capabilities was the founding of the first UK Cochrane Centre and later the National Health Service (NHS) Centre for Reviews and Dissemination, in York. At the time of writing, the Cochrane Collaboration has published more than 4,500 systematic reviews and is now widely recognized in the field of medicine. In 1991 the research and development strategy of the NHS and Department of Health laid out the foundations for evidence-based practice by articulating a new relationship between basic and applied research, and between the research and clinical communities. A key aspect of the program was the 1992 establishment of the UK Cochrane Centre at Oxford under the leadership of Sir Iain Chalmers and the founding of the Cochrane Collaboration in 1993.

In terms of significant knock-on effects for social work, a decisive moment came in 1999 with an exploratory meeting at University College London. The meeting was attended by several contributors to the Cochrane Collaboration (C1), and resulted in the establishment of an international steering group for the Campbell Collaboration (C2). The meeting agreed that an international collaboration, called the Campbell Collaboration, be required to prepare and maintain systematic reviews of research on the effects of interventions in areas such as education, criminal justice, and social policy and social care (Boruch *et al.* 2004). In particular, this meeting was keen to explore the extent to which the medical model of the C1 could be extended and reproduced in other fields, including social work, criminal justice and education. The intent was to understand whether and how well the C1's standards and protocols in medicine might be adapted to the proposed C2 focus.[5] This was considered essential in establishing the way in which Cochrane protocols could be adapted to systematic reviews of studies of effects in social, educational and criminological interventions. Funding for the meeting was provided by the NHS Research and Development Programme, the Department for Education and Employment and the Teacher Training Agency. The list of attendees of the first meeting, chaired by Iain Chalmers, is a veritable Who's Who of 'effectiveness-minded researchers', many of whom went on to champion evidence-based practice in their various home institutions and disciplinary fields, including Geraldine Macdonald (University of Bristol), Ian Sinclair (University of York), Kathy Sylva (University of Oxford), Teresa Smith (University of Oxford), Ron Feldman (Columbia University), Ann Oakley (Institute of Education, London), Phil Davies (British Cabinet Office and Oxford University), Judy Sebba (Department for Education and Employment) and David Gough (Institute of Education). The minutes noted that Brian Sheldon (Centre for Evidence Based Social Services) (see below) was unable to attend but wished to be kept informed. In 2000 a further progress meeting, attended by Chalmers and Macdonald, announced that the US Department of Education's Office of Planning and Evaluation, under the direction of Alan Ginsburg, had invested monies in the Campbell Collaboration.[6]

Apart from attracting the attendance of notable evidence-based supporters, we may ask why this scoping meeting for the Campbell Collaboration was so crucial in laying the foundations for an evidence-based social work. The meeting minutes and comments reported are revealing in this respect. Macdonald (1999c: 5) presented a paper on a 'systematic review of the effects of day care for pre-school children'. Having systematically searched journals and other sources and checked 920 studies or abstracts identified through this search, eight RCTs, measuring a wide range of outcomes, were selected for inclusion in this review.[7] For her presentation, Oakley (1999: 7) 'noted that randomized controlled trials and other forms of experimentation can, and should, be undertaken in social and educational research' but recognized that with social sciences 'only a small proportion of its output consists of randomized controlled trials' (see section below on hardening the evidence network). The proposed collaboration on social and educational interventions would, therefore, 'confront a proportionately larger literature on non-randomized and poorly controlled evidence' (*ibid.*: 7). Judy Sebba (1999: 11) presented a paper that called for 'more randomized controlled trials, systematic reviews and meta-analyses; better use of available randomized controlled trials, systematic reviews and meta-analyses; the development of a hierarchy of evidence covering all of these; and acceptance of systematic reviews within the UK Research Assessment Exercise'.

The differences between the three presentations are indicative of core issues that have plagued the evidence-based practice debate in social work. From the minutes, Macdonald's and Sebba's presentations appear to be uncritical, illustrative of 'what works' and 'how to do it'. As such, it is simply a practical matter of adopting and translating the medical epistemology of evidence and its infrastructure across to the social sciences in a normative, procedural and functionalist manner. Oakley's paper, on the other hand, while accepting the virtues of RCTs, is critical and challenging about the comparative research agenda. In actor network terms, Macdonald's is an implementation narrative that is illustrative of 'blackboxing', whereby the assumption is that the evidence-based epistemology is stable, i.e., that its underlying structure and methodology are unquestionable. Blackboxing is a sub-process of network formation in which complexity is reduced and simplified by treating the object, in this case systematic reviews, as having a pre-disposed legitimacy. With blackboxing, the legitimacy of scientific research is assumed to be obvious, or 'natural', in order to achieve an effect, namely, to curb opposition or alternatives. Sebba's narrative is a further example of blackboxing but it is also illustrative of what actor network theorists refer to as 'boundary work'. With Sebba, we see how evidence and its concomitant terms are constructed as a boundary object, whereby it is a development that inhabits several research communities – e.g., medicine, nursing and education – but is forced to satisfy the informational requirements of each in the same uniform way. Evidence is an object that is forced to travel across disciplinary borders and maintain the same sort of constant identity. As a boundary object, evidence must be 'plastic' enough to adapt to the local needs of the Campbell group but robust enough to maintain a common identity across C1 and C2 sites. As Bowker and Leigh Starr (1999: 297) note, 'Such objects have different meanings in different social worlds but their structure is common enough to more than one world to make them recognizable, a means of translation'. We can see here that Sebba is construing 'commonality' as advantageous in managing 'evidence' as boundary work and installing it as coherent across intersecting communities. This is a key bridging tactic in translating the Cochrane medicine-based approach across to the Campbell social sciences agenda, which involves mobility, stability and combinability of evidence. Oakley's presentation, while still advocating the emergent evidence-based practice agenda, is a critical reflection on the relation between medical and social sciences. If the Macdonald and Sebba contributions were representative of a straightforward adoption of evidence-based practice, for social work and education respectively, then Oakley's would be indicative of what we might call culturally sensitive practices advocating a more nuanced adaptation strategy. A question raised at the meeting focused on the status of non-randomized controlled trials, and how they fit in with RCTs in establishing best evidence, especially given that there may be more non-randomized than randomized trials in the social sciences. 'It was noted that the situation had been similar in health care but there had been a quantum leap in the number and quality of randomized trials since the 1950s, especially during the 1980s and 1990s' (*ibid.*: 8). The boundary object justification around RCTs is clear: if only social sciences would follow the lead of the medical sciences, they too could see the same miraculous leap in RCTs. Similarly, the value of theoretical thinking is narrowly defined to adjust to the requirements of the 'what works' agenda. It was noted at the meeting that while 'acknowledging that theory is important in scientific inquiry, it was stressed that this needs to be related to problems and problem solving' (*ibid.*: 8). Irreversibility is not a problem and we see the hegemony of the Cochrane (C1) translation process – as the weaving together of key evidence-based practice components – bringing previously unconnected elements into an alignment for the prototype Campbell Collaboration, later morphed as C2.

The feedback in the minutes of the Social Work and Social Care Discussion Group is particularly revealing in strategically positioning this cohort within the emerging evidence-based network:

> People in this group felt that although there was a good representation of participants from education and criminal justice, there was a need *for active networking* in the areas of social care and social policy. Members of this group expressed a willingness to take responsibility for developing such a network.
>
> (1999: 16, emphasis added)[8]

And so they did. The Social Work and Social Care Group mobilized itself around the mission of converting key stakeholders to the mantra of evidence-based practice. However, implicit here is the view that Social Work and Social Care were some way behind their counterparts in Education and Criminal Justice, both in terms of phased development and whole-hearted commitment to the project. In the group, some anxieties were raised about the relevance and applicability of evidence-based approaches to social work:

> Some concern was expressed about the methodological complexities of community or area-based interventions. It was recognized, however, that the social care and social policy network *would have to start somewhere*, and that it might be wise to begin by focusing on family and individual interventions and consider community based interventions later.
>
> (*ibid.*: 16, emphasis added)

What is revealing about this statement is not only that it confirms the psychologistic bias intrinsic to the evidence-based practice agenda, with the suggested focus on family and individual – behavioural – interventions rather than structural or ecological ones, but most strikingly it admits that a network would have 'to start somewhere'. As we saw in the discussion of diffusion theory in Chapter 4, this suggests a self-fulfilling prophecy at work, whereby it was considered a foregone conclusion that evidence-based initiatives had to happen irrespective of methodological quirks or professional resistance. Expectations were important features of the decision and impacted significantly on the later network formation.[9] Based on the success of the Cochrane Collaboration, the Campbell exploratory group was aware that once the translation process had been achieved, the innovation would follow a path from which it was difficult to diverge, becoming irreversible as protocols became firmly established.

Centre for Evidence-Based Social Services

The network formation of evidence-based social work that was later mobilized nationally had its embryonic roots in a small corner of England in places that many readers are unlikely to have heard of, such as Poole and Torbay. What is certain is that the enrolment strategies, agenda-setting and alliance formations around evidence-based practice initiated in this region, under the auspices of the Centre for Evidence-Based Social Services (CEBSS), had significant knock-on effects for the way the evidence-based agenda was rolled out in UK social work. The boundaries between research, evaluation and advocacy were unclear and, in some key respects, the Centre effectively became a campaigning and lobbying group for the virtues of evidence-based practice. While other evidence-based organizations, such as Research in Practice and Making Research Count, had an important influence, CEBSS was by far the most vociferous and partisan. Lovelock *et al.* (2004) describe the manoeuvring of CEBSS at the time of its inception in 1997 as a type of 'gladiatorial positioning' and one that was opposed by the wider social work research community. CEBSS was funded by a consortium of local authorities and the Department of Health, to the tune of £2.5 million. From its inception, it was very obvious that CEBSS at Exeter was on a mission, championed by its charismatic leader, Brian Sheldon. The multi-talented Sheldon was an organizer, entrepreneur, strategist, researcher and public relations man, having the ability to pass from one role to another and play them all with equal delight. Sheldon's ambition was to transform British social work, to make it pass from relying on interpretive judgement to evidence-based decisions and, more ambitiously, to engineer an 'evidence-based society'. His was a key intervention in the translation process that began to gather momentum in British social work.

Surprisingly, given the amount of strategic investment from the Department of Health, only two substantial publications came out of the tightly formed CEBSS group and none by top-tier publishers. The first was Sheldon and Chilvers' *Evidence-based social care: a study of prospects and problems*, in 2000. The second only appeared in 2005, as *Evidence-based social work: a guide for the perplexed*. This do-it-yourself guide was written by Newman, Moseley, Tierney and Ellis. Lead author Tony Newman worked for Barnardo's as research officer and had written three modular-type books on 'what works', with various client groups. Between 1999 and 2005, this CEBSS/Barnardo's alliance that joined evidence-based practice with the controversial 'what works' agenda in social care held firm. The CEBSS team, including Sheldon, Chilvers, Ellis, Moseley and Tierney, did get together in 2004 to write 'An empirical study of the obstacles to evidence-based practice', a chapter for Andy Bilson's *Evidence-based practice and social work*. The capacity-building and leverage activities of CEBSS focused mainly on the southwest of England, working in collaboration with local authority social services departments and voluntary agencies, particularly Barnardo's. Indeed, the main research activities of CEBSS, other than its surveys on the uptake of evidence-based practice in practice contexts, centred on commissioning small-scale, locally based evaluations with a definite preference for evaluative studies that would focus on RCTs.

Despite the few quality publications, there was a definite religious zeal about the way in which CEBSS went about its business and some may consider a propagandist ideology in its activities, video productions and newsletter publications. Rallying calls relayed to potential converts through the CEBSS Newsletter (1999: 2)[10] were explicit about the radical nature of the mission: 'The clearest message we have from studies of research usage [as can be seen in this issue of the Newsletter] is that attempts to bring about a cultural change are first a matter of setting up a debate in the hope of changing hearts and minds'. Isn't evidence-based practice supposed to be against opinion-driven sentiment and, more reasonably, wouldn't the evidence itself suffice to make the case? At the time, Sheldon and his associates were clearly impatient, dismayed by the slow speed of change and fed up with the resistance they met within social work. If the evidence-based practice revolution were stumbling, a clarion call to the masses would be necessary. This is how Sheldon described the situation in 1999:

> 'Oil tankers and tug boats' about sums up the mechanics of this problem of bringing research and practice closer together. Our only comfort is that in CEBSS we have at least the advantage of regular communication with captains and navigators as well as with crews regarding course heading, and the known position of shoals and rocks!
>
> (CEBSS Newsletter, Number 4, 1999: 1)

What is striking about this piece is that Sheldon has no awareness that the ship might never reach its destination. The proselytizing in the CEBSS Newsletter often fell short of the rigour, objectivity and integrity that are claimed for evidence-based practice by those who champion it. In reviewing one of the authors' articles that appeared in the *British Journal of Social Work*, which later became one of the most cited social work articles on evidence-based practice, the editor dismissively rebutted it by claiming: 'An interesting article (though, ahem, profoundly mistaken) on why evidence-based practice is a bad idea. We have invited Webb to take part in our Spotlight conference (see front page) 'cos that's just the kind of folk we are (sadists)' (CEBSS Newsletter, Number 9, 2001: 3).

So much for Macdonald's plea for more systematic and 'considered views'. And yet, several years after the debate in the *British Journal of Social Work* on the validity of evidence-based practice, Sheldon appeared haunted by the earlier debate and doggedly returned to the same theme in a keynote address at Liverpool John Moore's university in 2007, with a paper entitled 'The validity of evidence based practice in social work'. Sheldon used the last issue of the CEBSS Newsletter (2004), provocatively entitled 'A triumph of hope over experience', for his swansong. Here he abundantly demonstrated his frustrations at the resistance to the uptake of evidence-based practice in social work. In contrasting the successes of evidence-based practice in healthcare against social work, he exclaims:

> But then, they had, and have the money; the technical backup, and the benefit of not having been educated by sociologists who have never interviewed an

up-against-it client in their lives, and who would rather have been sitting on the Rive Gauche in black jumpers, glancing at slim volumes of post-modernist nonsense.

(CEBSS Newsletter, Number 16, 2004: 1)

Some may consider this remonstration a form of narrow partisanship from a man who swears by experimental objectivity and RCTs. In the same CEBSS Newsletter, Sheldon (2004: 2) worries about the 'the enemy of progress towards evidence-based practice' and the subtitle of a photograph of Sheldon with his associates states 'A typical CEBSS "seizing power" meeting'. Heady stuff, and clearly this outfit meant business. The belief was that it is here in this provincial English city, in the heart of this united and versatile team, that evidence-based practice will take shape. It seems that the message, which was hammered out day after day, is simple: evidence-based social work is the future, casework is barely trying to survive and a randomized controlled social work is for tomorrow. Sheldon was particularly keen on cohorting, mentoring and coaching his immediate team. As Akrich, Callon and Latour (2002a: 212) maintain, 'It is because the form of a technical object [EBP] is directly dependent upon the identity of the actors who participate [the CEBSS 'power-seizing' team] in its development and the nature of the relations which they maintain'. But, rather confusingly, in the final paragraph of his introduction to the Newsletter, Sheldon announces his retirement from CEBSS to work on his joint-authored textbook, *A textbook of social work* for Routledge (with Geraldine Macdonald, who was also Visiting Professor at CEBSS), and says: 'Note that the phrase "evidence based" is not in the title, because we think it time to just *assume* this principle'. The smell of victory at last! (See Chapter 1, where we note that the case for or against evidence-based practice needs to be argued rather than assumed.) CEBSS ceased operations on 31 October 2004. Meanwhile, the Research in Practice (RIP) evidence-based group, has collected archival material of its newsletters, reports, video-clips and research skills modules on its website (http://www.rip.org.uk/).

CEBSS is a good example of how, if we are to explain the development of evidence-based practice in the UK, concepts from actor network theory are extremely helpful. It demonstrates the collective dimension of the emergence of evidence-based practice and, as we shall see, shows how the process of adoption is synonymous with adaptation in the UK. For the analysis of CEBSS, two actor network concepts are particularly pertinent in articulating the network activities: *interessement* and *enrolment*. The Centre is a rich instance of what Callon (1986) calls a 'model of *interessement*', whereby the fate of the innovation – in this case, evidence-based practice – depends on the active participation of all those who have decided to develop it. It was an arena where alliances were formed, strengthening the shifting and fragmentary networks with each other and with the external agencies. *Interessement* is best regarded as a process of legitimation, whereby CEBSS attempted to convince practitioners and managers in social work to accept that the evidence-based practice agenda was compatible with their own interests and to convey how such joint interests could create incentives that would bind the partnerships together. With CEBSS, these activities went beyond traditional research agendas, as with the 'hearts and minds' campaign, to include business communities, frontline practitioners and political actors (national policy-makers and civil servants) and co-opted 'international stars' from evidence-led institutions, such as the Cochrane and Campbell Collaborations. A key feature of the distinctive regionalist strategy, adopted by CEBSS to maximize a concentrated effort – with its partnerships, local commissions and community engagements – was characterized by the personal chemistry, albeit bounded by codes of professionalism, between the director, the research assistants and external stakeholders, particularly Barnardo's and local social services departments in Avon, Somerset, Devon and Wiltshire. CEBSS was particularly prone to co-opting groups and individuals in the pursuit of collective objectives. The southwest of England university axis – between the universities of Exeter, Bristol and Bath – was also significant in this respect.

Flying high with SCIE

The Social Care Institute for Excellence (SCIE) was established by the UK government in 2001 to improve social care services. The strategic ambition was to model it on the National Institute for Clinical Excellence (NICE) in medicine, set up in 1999.[11] We have seen that mobilization for action is a particularly important strategy in the formalization of evidence-based practice, especially when driven by determined charismatic leaders. The appointment of Ray Jones in 2001 as the first chief executive of SCIE was no exception to this rule. Prior to the SCIE post, he had been director of Wiltshire Social Services (in the southwest) since 1992 and later became chairman of the British Association of Social Workers (BASW).

As a close associate of Sheldon, Jones had been involved with CEBSS from its inception in 1996. Sheldon had been instrumental in Jones's obtaining his Visiting Professorship at Exeter. In announcing his new role as CEO of SCIE in the CEBSS Newsletter, Jones stated that 'SCIE's task, in partnership with others (which will certainly include CEBSS), is to collate, translate and disseminate evidence of "what works" in social care' (CEBSS Newsletter, Number 10, 2001: 7). In the CEBSS Newsletter, Jones further stated that 'CEBSS, along with other organisations such as *Research in Practice* and *Making Research Count*, has helped to pioneer the way in social care to ensure that we learn from, and act on, the evidence of "what works – for whom, how and why"' (*ibid.*).[12]

In 2002 Jones quit as chief executive of SCIE after only seven months, due to a dispute over his contract. Following this, he resumed his post as director of adult and community services at Wiltshire County Council. However, in 2006 he also quit that position after cost savings were forced on the council by the NHS funding crisis and, in the same year, he stepped down from the chair of the BASW, citing a clash between himself and the BASW's chief executive, Ian Johnston, for the reason behind his resignation. Another key actor in the early SCIE appointments was Mike Fisher, Director of Research and Reviews, responsible for the important and powerful role of developing knowledge reviews. It is likely that he was enlisted to firm up and initiate various evidence-based positions from a research perspective. In this capacity, Fisher co-authored (with P. Marsh, in 2005) *Developing the evidence base for social work and social care practice* (SCIE, Report 10, 2005) and (with E. Coran, in 2006) *The conduct of systematic research reviews for SCIE knowledge reviews.* He had previously worked with Geraldine Macdonald at the University of Bristol and she was elected to the SCIE Board of Trustees when it began its operations in 2001. Consolidating her position, Macdonald was also appointed as Business Director of Information and Knowledge Management at the Commission for Social Care Inspection, chaired by Denise Platt in 2004 (see section below).

To set up SCIE and appoint the right champions, spokespersons and inter-mediaries is not only to give oneself the means with which to specify the UK evidence-based agenda; it is, above and before all, to put oneself in a position to formalize that agenda by carefully mobilizing and translating particular types of evidence-based initiatives. The commitment of Fisher, Jones and others such as Amanda Edwards and Jane Campbell, along with Macdonald, to building the evidence-based empire and trying to colonize traditional social work practice, through the auspices of SCIE, is self-evident. The way in which they intended to pull this off, however, required some nifty manoeuvrings and careful tactical thinking. It was the fruit of a strategic calculation. SCIE had always been acutely aware of the necessity of measures to evaluate its impact, and its image with the consumer was paramount. In the early days of its operations, SCIE was very careful not to display its evidence-based credentials or aspirations. In some respects, it seemed that it wanted to distance itself from organizations like CEBSS, initially wishing to co-opt or contain oppositional tendencies in the social work research community. While there was an alignment with the mission of CEBSS and a convergence around core principles of articulating what was considered best practice social work, there was also a displacement at work. The tactic of accommodating resistance is a fairly standard one and reminds us of the way in which medical psychiatry neutralized the anti-psychiatry movement by co-opting key concepts into the project, thereby blunting opposition. It can also be viewed as a more subtle mechanism of trying to encourage dissenters to put aside differences in order to maintain the evidence network and thus to conform. It is readily apparent that the network logic of SCIE is entirely different from that of CEBSS. From the actor network perspective, SCIE can be seen as a mechanism to 'smooth the path' for the national deployment of the evidence-based agenda that articulated a more subtle approach than CEBSS in attempting to ensure effective and amicable communication between stakeholders. It is worth examining some of the SCIE products to identify the way in which the evidence-based agenda is being rolled out in the UK.

Knowledge reviews

More recently, knowledge reviews have been identified as being of central impor-tance by SCIE in enabling social work research to facilitate the hardening of the evidence-based policy and practice agenda. They are defined by SCIE as taking 'a systematic approach to the gathering, analysis and appraisal of knowledge on a particular topic. They describe the material available, the evidence that emerges and the findings drawn from the evidence.' SCIE knowledge reviews are not reducible to systematic reviews, since their broader remit comprises several elements in combining a research knowledge gathered in a research review – a version of the systematic review methodology – and practice knowledge assembled through a practice survey.

The authors of *SCIE Knowledge Review 7* stipulate that 'Evidence-informed policy and practice demands increasing recourse to research as a key source of knowledge about how to improve practice' (Walter *et al.* 2004: v). SCIE states that 'the most trustworthy knowledge comes from systematic reviews where we look at a whole body of work on a given topic' (Luckock *et al.* 2006: 2).[13] It is likely that when the source of knowledge is not perceived as trustworthy, knowledge transfer can be expected to be a difficult task. However, it is fallacious to talk about trustworthy knowledge, since no research paradigm can guarantee this moral claim. Instead of making claims for certain objective knowledge, SCIE wishes to trade on the notion of 'trustworthy knowledge', by which they mean that which is genuinely believed, for good reasons, by colleagues and the research community. This becomes a matter of trusting the source of the knowledge, and assessing values, meanings and beliefs, and not the instrumental usage of trust given by SCIE. As Daukas (2007: 24) states, 'Epistemic trustworthiness is defined as a complex character state that supervenes on a relation between first- and second-order beliefs, including beliefs about others as epistemic agents'.

Thus trustworthiness is an acquired attribute of social actors involved in networked relationships and not an objective measure of systematic reviews or deductive reasoning. It strikes us that rather than using the subjectively loaded notion of trustworthy research, the concept of 'fitness for purpose' is much better as the appropriate measure of quality, meaning that the science should be methodologically good enough for weight to be attached to it in informing various practice contexts. What is most evident from the systematic review work thus far undertaken in social work is that they tend to reach uncertain conclusions. Moreover, they are often unable to provide specific guidance on effective – or even ineffective – interventions. Instead, they tend to conclude with statements such as 'good evidence is currently lacking' or that 'most results were statistically non-significant'. There appears to be little room for specific recommendations and instead a tendency for broad brush-stroke generalizations. Although this may be an accurate representation of the state of the evidence, it is not useful for guiding practice or policy for little evidence exists to allow the frontline practice issues to be answered. What does this tell us? (i) Quite simply, few relevant outcome evaluations – randomized, controlled or otherwise – of social work have been carried out; (ii) as a methodology, systematic review work does not appropriately lend itself to complex social problems and issues intrinsic to social work; and (iii) standardization of practice is the underlining ambition of these technologies.

In the following snapshot analysis, we draw attention to some significant problems associated with knowledge reviews, focusing particularly on search criteria and definitional issues. Search criteria are a contentious process, with opposing schools of thought with regard to critical issues surrounding study selection. The debate that centres on the selection process is important, because the inclusion and exclusion of studies determines the scope and validity of systematic review results. It also determines the amount of bias in the outcomes. Moreover, if the constituent problem formulation and selection criteria were flawed, the review's conclusions would be equally flawed, a principle known as 'garbage in, garbage out'. In *SCIE Knowledge Review 18* (Marchant *et al.* 2007: 4), 'Necessary stuff: the social care needs of children with complex health care needs and their families', the authors acknowledge some significant problems associated with the methodology:

> Definitional problems related to the key concepts of this review besieged the team from the start. We struggled with terminology at all levels: in our own discussions, in keywording for the research review, in our contacts with children and families and in our approach to different professionals.

With *SCIE Knowledge Review 16* (Fauth and Mahdon 2007), 'Improving social and health care services', the aim was to explore the processes and actions that have proven most effective in bringing about and sustaining improvement in social and healthcare services. The search criteria for the research review focused on organizational change, and improvement is inclusive of the various stages of organizational change including planning, implementation and evaluation. Here we may identify a very common problem that emerges in systematic reviews around selecting inclusion and exclusion criteria:

> The authors report that 'the project team brainstormed the following primary keywords, which were approved by SCIE' included: organisational change; organisational development; organisational transformation; organisational improvement; organisational learning; change process; and (whole) systems change.
>
> (Fauth and Mahdon 2007: 10)

First, at very basic level, the search results will vary significantly depending on whether the key Americanized 'organization' or Anglophile 'organisation' term is used. Moreover, there are some very important search terms that are missing from the list that would have significantly contributed to the search findings and the evaluative analysis. If we are right, this suggests that the selected criterion of key terms approved by SCIE is biased. It is acknowledged that broad iterative literature searches can assist in problem formulation, so we undertook a rough and ready search using features of Google to highlight the deficiencies in the keyword search for *SCIE Knowledge Review 18* (Marchant *et al.* 2007). The most obvious important terms excluded are: 'organisational culture' and 'organisational theory'. Others are 'organisational behaviour', 'organisational systems' and 'organisational dissent'. Figure 5.1 gives the number of Google search hits, to demonstrate the varying significance of each of these terms.

It is apparent that the authors of *SCIE Knowledge Review 18* (Marchant *et al.* 2007) did not seek out established theoretical frameworks from relevant fields to provide structure to the problem formulation and data analysis stages of the research. If they had done so, a very productive and cutting-edge field would have emerged, referred to as 'critical management studies' in the organizational studies literature. We find, for example, that Google Scholar produces 3,100,000 hits for 'critical management studies'. In this sense, the SCIE authors fall short of the requirements of what Ray Pawson (2006: 82) calls 'realist reviews', whereby the decisive aspects of a range of program theories are located, allowing the reviewer to pass into the 'inner workings of a programme and establish programme re-engineering as the potential goal' (see Chapter 3). The results of a realist review, advocated by Pawson (2006), combine theoretical understanding and empirical evidence, and focus on explaining the relationship between the context in which the intervention is applied, the mechanisms by which it works and the outcomes which are produced. Unlike the reviews commissioned by SCIE, the realist review strategy will not tell policy-makers or managers 'what works' or not but it will 'provide the policy and practice community with the kind of rich, detailed and highly practical understanding of complex social interventions which is likely to be of much more use to them when planning and implementing programmes at a national, regional or local level' (Pawson *et al.* 2005: 21).

SCIE as a translation agency

Drawing on Latour's characterization of modernity, we can evaluate SCIE in terms of two interlocking formalization practices: those of 'purification' and 'hybridization'. In the translation process, SCIE creates mixtures between types of method that aim to formalize evidence-based social work by a process of enculturation whereby they try to achieve credibility by stabilizing the policy initiatives and methods in the evidence network.[14] The broad ambition of SCIE within the UK, and increasingly on an international scale, is to produce evidence-based networks that connect seemingly disparate elements into an organizational thread. In rhetorical terms, the clean construction or purification process begins with devices, such as

---

Organisational culture

A Google search for organisational culture reveals 1,670,000 hits; Google Scholar, 1,090,000; Google Advanced Search, 1,590,000.

Organisational theory

Organisational behaviour on Google, 7,310,000; Google Scholar, 300,000; Google Advanced Search, 515,000.

Organisational dissent on Google, 585,000; Google Scholar, 54,600

Organisational systems on Google, 4,650,000; Google Scholar, 1,340,000; Google Advanced Search, 190,000.

Figure 5.1 Google search hits.

with the SCIE mission statement about what they do: 'capture and co-produce knowledge about good practice' and 'communicate knowledge, evidence and innovation'. In constructing the concepts – the tools of description – in one continuous chain as they apply to social work – knowledge, capture, co-produce, communicate and evidence – they are conveyed as normative, straightforward and unproblematic. In this sense, SCIE is performing as a translation agency in a very similar way to traditional scientific research laboratories. As Crawford (in Ritzer 2004: 1) notes for proponents of actor network theory, 'the "success" of science is attributable to the ability of scientific networks: to force entities to pass through labs or clinics in order to harness "scientific evidence" within disputes; to translate materials, actors, and texts into *inscriptions* that allow influence at a distance'. We can see this process at play in the activities of SCIE and may also observe how it has become what Latour calls a 'centre of translation', where network elements are defined and controlled, and strategies for translation – knowledge reviews, practice guides, research briefings, resource guides and activity reports – are developed and considered. SCIE is engaged in the stabilization and reproduction of the evidence network at the behest of others, but most importantly in the construction and maintenance of the network of evidence-based social work in the UK. The strategic aim of SCIE is the formalization of evidence-based knowledge and artefacts, which, across time, are translated as a network becomes more extensive and/or concentrated, and as subsequent iterations emerge the formalization process is hardened.

Barnett House, Oxford: from reformism to rapprochement?

Up until 2003, Barnett House at the University of Oxford was one of the most prestigious and established training centres for social work.[15] Founded in 1913, it was a centre for social studies in the inter-war years and one of the UK's first centres for social work training which began at Oxford University in 1913 and was formally established at Barnett House in 1946.

In 1974 the Diploma in Social and Administrative Studies was replaced by the MSc in Applied Social Studies, a two-year graduate degree combining the old diploma and professional training, and attracting twenty-five to thirty candidates each year. However, in 2003 the social work professional training program at Barnett House was discontinued after running successfully for some ninety years. In 2003 a new postgraduate course in Evidence-based Social Work was successfully launched with an initial international intake of twenty students. To capture a wider audience, this was later renamed MSc in Evidence-based Social Intervention. One key difference is that this is increasingly in an international setting, with the majority of graduate students at Barnett House now from outside the UK. The program details say that there is a particular emphasis on quantitative methods, especially appraisal and design of RCTs, and systematic reviews, and their application to social interventions. In line with these curriculum developments, the Oxford department established the Centre for Evidence Based Intervention (CEBI) to evaluate interventions for social and psychosocial problems, in particular through conducting RCTs, systematic reviews and other evaluation designs.

The key figures at the new Oxford CEBI Group are Paul Montgomery and Frances Gardner, who are both clinical psychologists by background and well-versed in experimental methodologies. The Oxford Group has closely aligned itself with the Cochrane (C1) and Campbell (C2) Collaborations. A quick glance at the research outputs shows the saturation of RCT interventions and systematic reviews.[16] To give a flavour of the emphasis: 'Randomised trial of a media-based parenting intervention'; 'Randomised trial of self-help intervention and melatonin for sleep problems in the elderly'; 'Early family-based prevention of risk for drug abuse: a randomized controlled trial'; 'A family-based prevention for early conduct problems: randomized controlled trial'; 'A series of systematic reviews of effectiveness of interventions following physical abuse'; and 'A series of systematic reviews of personal care'. The site lists thirty-two systematic reviews carried out by members of CEBI for C1 and C2.

The Oxford example demonstrates a remarkable turnaround in events for mainstream social work training. Clearly for Oxford the new options were more economically attractive with the recruitment of international students. Moreover, professional training courses are notoriously resource intensive and expensive to run, but to abandon a long tradition of social work education at Oxford is not only indicative of strategic disinvestment but, most importantly, a sea-change in fortunes for evidence-based practice. If the formalization agenda for evidence-based practice needed an academically esteemed endorsement, what could be more powerful than the dreaming spires of Oxford? It is self-evident that endorsements from powerful institutional constituents improve evidence-based practice's chances of success, signalling its reliability and trustworthiness, while facilitating legitimacy from consumers, prospective sponsoring and partner organizations, the general public, and government. The diffusion of the evidence network is also reliant on inter-organizational arrangements to leverage its reputation. Inter-organizational exchange relationships, such as those tight links between the Oxford CEBI and C1, act as endorsements that influence perceptions of the quality of evidence-based practice when unambiguous measures of quality do not exist or cannot be observed. It is important to remember at this point that the challenge of formalization processes of these infrastructure systems is that they become blackboxed for all those closely involved; their rationale and outputs are taken for granted.

The Platt Review: hardening the evidence-based agenda

Dame Denise Platt was commissioned by the UK Secretary of State to review *The status of social care* and her work was completed in April 2007. Her covering letter to Ivan Lewis, Parliamentary Under Secretary of State for Care Services, Department of Health, states that she 'hopes this report provides some ideas about how the service can begin to rebuild its confidence and the confidence of the public in the valuable, and for the most part, invisible service – social care' (2007b: 1). In fact, the tone of the review is indicative of the 'three strikes and you're out'[17] mentality and clearly signals that social care had jolly well better get its act together or else! Indeed, in April 2007, the Secretary of State announced that SCIE would be required to create a new system by the end of the year for identifying and disseminating evidence-based social work.

In order to understand the impact of the Platt Review in actor network terms, some background information is helpful. Dame Platt has been around the block a few times in her public sector management career. She graduated in economics and began a long career in the social services at Middlesex Hospital. Between 1986 and 1994, as director of social services for the London Borough of Hammersmith and Fulham, she had to pick up the debris left by the Tories. She was made a Dame in the Queen's Birthday Honours in June 2004. Platt has not published widely, which is unsurprising given all her directing, inspecting and governance activities. In 1992 she wrote 'Contracting and agreements with the voluntary sector: an SSD view' for the edited collection *Purchasing and providing social services in the 1990s: drawing the line* (Platt 1992), and in 1996 she published for the British Association of Social Workers under the strangely Leninist title *Then ... Now ... Onwards*. In 2002 Platt's 'Guidance on the single assessment process for older people; [and] guidance for local implementation' was published for a local authority. In 2007 she published 'Advice to care home operators on strategies for successful outcomes of social care inspections' in the *Journal of Care Services Management* (Platt 2007a). We do know that Platt very clearly believes in the mantra that some things work and others do not. In 2004 Platt, in her role as chair of the Commission for Social Care Inspection, warned that too many authorities were also coasting on one star, instead of aiming for excellence. In 2005 she was involved in launching the Bournemouth University publication, *Making it work: supporting workforce development across the social care sector*. She played a significant role in the drive for performance assessment benchmarking and the league table star-rating indicators for UK social services departments. In May 2006 she chaired a seminar, Creative Commissioning for Personalised Care, for the Commission for Social Care Inspection. The common underlying themes with this 'what works' literature by Platt are: contracting, commissioning, inspection, performance and quality audit. In other words, hardcore 'public sector managerialism'. The incessant drive to improve efficiencies and accountability across the workforce is clearly at stake with the Platt agenda. It could be argued that this is best understood in terms of control and regulation, not efficiencies and evidence.

From an actor network perspective, what is most interesting is the way Platt lambasted SCIE, chief among her targets, along with other notable social work institutions, such as the *British Journal of Social Work*. Her sharpest criticisms were reserved for the way in which SCIE had failed to replicate the promise of the evidence-based medical agenda and the prescriptive, regulatory features of NICE. In fact, the Platt Review is a shoddy piece of thinking which was badly researched and failed to consult widely with important and respected stakeholders. Nonetheless, as we shall see, the rhetoric has had a significant impact on pushing the evidence-based agenda in social work in a particular direction. Indeed, Platt's is a striking example of an intervention that is not based on any evidence in trying to force the evidence-based agenda.

Platt (2007b: 15) claimed that SCIE has disappointed the sector by failing adequately to fulfil its brief to disseminate good practice. 'There is widespread agreement that more is required than just making the material available', she observes, somewhat caustically. Platt went on to say that SCIE, now under new leadership, will be tasked with producing by the end of the year a fresh strategy for identification and dissemination of excellence. Her main criticisms (Platt 2007b: 13–17) about the failure of SCIE in fulfilling its mandate are summarized below:

•   The SCIE program is not perceived by top managers in the independent sector to have sufficient prestige to attract existing and aspiring leaders from across all three sectors of social care, as it does not include enough input from business.
•   Most people consider that a more effective dissemination strategy of 'what works' is needed. Increasing the capacity of the sector to make good use of research findings is perceived as a critical area for immediate development.
•   Dissemination of 'what works' was a prime reason for the creation of SCIE. There is disappointment in the sector that this function has not yet been effectively delivered for adult social care. Quicker progress on dissemination of good practice was expected. There is widespread agreement that more is required than just making the material available.

The managerialist intent is most apparent in the deliberations of Dame Platt and here we can detect why critics of evidence-based practice have warned that the methodology readily lends itself with an alignment to risk-management regimes and economic–political control. We noted above that establishing the evidence-based network in social work involves the enrolment of agencies and actors, i.e., coordinating roles that lead to the establishment of a stable network of alliances. We also mentioned that for enrolment to be successful, it requires others to yield – in this case, through the rhetoric of Platt, it is SCIE that must yield. That quality control, systems regulation, network alliance and the hardening of a narrow medical model version for SCIE figured centrally in the considerations of Platt is evidenced in the recommendations, endorsed by David Behan, Department of Health director general for social care, that: (i) SCIE should develop a closer relationship with the Care Services Improvement Partnership (CSIP) to agree priorities for service development, taking account of both research and inspection findings, and assist the service to take on board best practice; (ii) SCIE should be encouraged to give a higher profile to its dissemination role, particularly in respect of adult social care. Platt says that 'The National Institute for Health and Clinical Excellence (NICE) is valued for the guidance it gives to the service. It is also valued for what it tells the health service *not* to do because it is ineffective. Such advice [on what *not to do*] from SCIE would be similarly welcome' (Platt 2007b: 16). In affirming the negative, what is being recommended by Platt is not only the regulation and control of social work practice under the auspices of SCIE but also the 'one size fits all' standardization of that practice. That is, engineering a set of standard technical specifications for frontline practice that adhere to the evidence-based technology, with SCIE as the standardization agency in the process of ratifying, implementing and monitoring the standard.

The Platt Review has left a lasting impression on SCIE. Indeed, there has been a flurry of post-review activity at both SCIE and with the *British Journal of Social Work*.[18] In actor network terms, the Platt intervention maybe described as being part of the enrolment process whereby actors struggle to dominate the network-building. This is best considered as involving a tension between a defensive network (SCIE) and a more powerful challenging network (Platt, the Department of Health and government ministers). That the Platt Review rattled the executive officers of SCIE is most apparent in an examination of the SCIE Board meeting minutes from July 2007 onwards. At the 5 July meeting, Amanda Edwards, Acting CEO, introduced the item 'Review of the status of social care' and since that time it has become a standing agenda item for the Board. The minutes state that 'The Board strongly felt that the report on the Status of Social Care presented *a very significant opportunity* for SCIE and the social care sector to improve the service provided to users of social care and influence national policy' (SCIE 2007c: 2, emphasis added).[19] A 'significant opportunity', in committee-speak, is often another way of saying 'our back's to the wall, but let's put a positive spin on things'. Nevertheless, it reveals an uncritical compliance at the core of SCIE in its failure to challenge the sloppy, unrepresentative meanderings of Platt. Most interestingly, the minute reports that 'SCIE is well placed to lead the development of a strategy for dissemination and *achieve a consensus on what will embed best practice*' (*ibid.*, emphasis added). For 'best practice' read evidence-based social work and, as discussed in Chapter 7, the dissemination strategy adopted by SCIE is based on a flawed normative expectation that 'best practice' will materialize in a more or less fixed set of locations – social work agencies or the behaviour of individual social workers – to be performed and remain durable. We show that 'best practice' notions such as this rest on the false assumption that there is a stable and unified body of knowledge in social work. That SCIE is best placed to achieve a consensus on embedding best practice is also doubtful. It seems to us that SCIE is increasingly regarded as an unrepresentative 'central regulatory care regime', with agencies and divisional teams very much at the periphery of strategic directions. As will be shown in Chapter 7, there is no consensus, either in the research community or in policy formulations, as to what constitutes or will embed best practice for social work. Moreover, the dissemination attempts are often diluted as they are implemented, resulting in a 'sedimented layering' of partially digested evidence-based guidelines.

To get a feel for the fallout of the Platt Review on SCIE and the hardening of the evidence-based social work agenda, it is worthwhile to reflect on some related developments. Following the Platt Review, Julie Jones was headhunted from the Conservative-run Westminster Council in London and appointed as new chief executive to SCIE in July 2007. In the *Guardian* interview, 'The rule of evidence', Jones worried about the credibility gap between SCIE and NICE. In wishing to display her newly discovered evidence-based credentials, she commented:

> The allegation often is that the *evidence* to support the argument for social care is not as robust as it is in other areas. That may be because there just hasn't been the investment in research and *evidence*-gathering that there has been in areas like health. The answer is that we have got to pull together all that we know in a way that is convincing, and *evidence* based, because only an *evidence* base gets you the credibility.
>
> (*Guardian*, Wednesday 28 March 2007: 5; emphasis added.)

The citing of 'evidence' four times in this press statement – with an additional three citations later in the same interview – and the implication of a 'rule of law' metaphor certainly convey a strong impression, indicative of future directions for SCIE. The simple logic of the message is that more resources equal more evidence, and more evidence means more credibility. As well as constructing that all-important evidence base, Jones stated that her priorities would include building network alliances with bodies like NICE. Following the Platt Review, SCIE, in line with NICE, quickly modified the lead principle on its website to emphasize that it strives to be '*Authoritative*: we ensure that there is good evidence from research and other reliable sources for what we say'[20] (emphasis added).

Hardening the evidence network

Some parallel developments can be read alongside these of SCIE that are indicative of the shifting agenda in social work. The announcement by John Denham, UK Secretary of State for Innovation, in October 2008, that the social care sector will have its own National Skills Academy, working alongside SCIE, is indicative of a dumbing-down of social work education away from university professional education towards low-level, administrative functional skills training sponsored by employers.[21] Similarly, the development of a new National Social Care Research Ethics Committee (SCREC), also endorsed by SCIE, as a risk management body, is indicative of an ever-increasing regulation under the name of 'ethics' in the social care sector. Under Jones's leadership, it is likely that the production and stabilization of evidence-based networks through standardized formats for best practice and knowledge reviews will remain at the core of SCIE's colonizing mission. Attempts to use the translation infrastructure to instil 'obligatory passage points', as the embedding of an evidence-based culture, in which all frontline practitioners must pass in order to execute an intervention, is the ultimate goal.

Moreover, it seems, there will be an increased emphasis for SCIE on conforming to wider network alliances of more powerful agencies, such as NICE and the Cochrane Collaboration, and enrolling new recruits, particularly senior executives from business and the independent sector. Chief executive Jones clearly wants to press home jurisdiction claims for a particular brand of evidence-based social work as a means of overcoming territorial disputes from allied professions, such as education, nursing or probation. In lieu of Platt, the overall SCIE strategy is indicative of territorial boundary claims, or what Andrew Abbott (1988) calls reclaims for 'professional jurisdiction' whereby intentional attempts are made to mark or delimit a territory – e.g., the network of evidence-based social work – to exert order and territorial control in a certain field of practice. Abbott remarks that a key factor which leaves professional bodies, such as SCIE, prone to external attack is the existence of a problem where no treatment can be inferred. To counteract this potential downfall, Abbott (1988: 50) suggested that professions often direct these unsolvable problems to elite consultants or have them clinically researched as 'crucial anomalies'. These procedures help to make the difficult problem connected with a vague public label, 'which serves as a stopgap against dangerous questioning' (*ibid.*: 51). With SCIE we may be witnessing a morphogenic structuring process, which Kärrholm (2007: 445) calls a 'territorial practice of power'. This process is described 'in terms of network stabilizations where connections between a set of actors or actants (e.g., rules and regulations, borders, subterritories, information technology, legal patents and mandates, expert behaviors, and norms) aim at increasing stability and predictability'.

Finally, it is important to mention the profile of three interrelated activities which, while not bearing directly on social work, represent a hardening of the institutional infrastructure for evidence-based practice in UK social sciences. These activities demonstrate the manner in which evidence-based practice is increasingly multi-disciplinary and bearing on a range of public sector dimensions. They also illustrate the way the actor network is being formed around evidence-based practice whereby 'translators' can be seen to build alliances around their definitions of the research world. First, the Economic and Social Research Council (ESRC), the UK's leading research and training agency addressing economic and social concerns, established the Evidence Network in 2001. This was developed on the basis of a decision in 1999 by the ESRC that a major initiative was needed to 'bring social science research much nearer to the decision making process'. Funding of £3 million over three years was allocated in 2000 for a national coordinating Centre for Evidence Policy and Practice and a network of research nodes that made up the initial Evidence Network. With further funding since 2003, the Network has grown substantially through the Centre's Associate program, and some 900 researchers, practitioners and policy-makers worldwide had joined by October 2007.[22] The Evidence Network replicates some of the earlier ambitions of CEBSS more broadly within the social sciences. Its mission is built 'around the belief that better quality decisions will be made in public and social policy if the process is informed by a good knowledge of the issue in hand' (*ibid.*). Second, and as part of its brief, the ESRC developed *Evidence & Policy: A Journal of Research, Debate and Practice* as the first international, peer-reviewed journal dedicated to exploring the relationship between research evidence, policy-making and practice. This evidence-based journal was founded by the Centre for Evidence & Policy in 2005, and is published by The Policy Press. The journal 'addresses the interests of those who plan and deliver public services, and those who provide the evidence base for their evaluation and development. Interdisciplinary in scope, it covers a wide range of social and public policy issues – from social care to education, from public health to criminal justice.'[23] Two leading champions of evidence-based practice in the UK – Amanda Edwards (from SCIE) and David Gough (from the Institute of Education, University of London) – are on the editorial management board of the journal. The third recent example of a hardening of the institutional infrastructure for evidence-based practice in the UK is offered by the powerful Evidence for Policy and Practice Information and Co-ordinating Centre (EPPI-Centre), which is part of the Social Science Research Unit at the Institute of Education, University of London. Established in 1993, EPPI describes its achievements as having been at 'the forefront of carrying out research synthesis and developing review methods in social science and public policy. We are dedicated to making reliable research findings accessible to the people who need them, whether they are making policy, practice or personal decisions.'[24] David Gough is also the director of EPPI and Ann Oakley, one of the fiercest advocates of evidence-based practice (see section above on the Campbell Collaboration), is the founding director. These developments in the UK help us to explain how, despite fragmentation of institutional sites and goals, it has been possible for the evidence-based program to build networks of resources around a particular articulation of methodology, implementation and practice intervention that increasingly become taken for granted. We have seen how a strategic convergence occurs with the main players in the evidence-based network, and how strategizing is a mode of accommodation of both possible converts and critics. Thus, as we shall see in the next chapter, the evidence-based strategy for social work exists to the extent that its materialization is made real by the network of organizational actors – human and non-human – that support it. In simple terms, through the research–policy interface evidence-based social work permits the possibility of narrowly prescribing for frontline practitioners 'what counts' as knowledge at the exclusion of other forms of knowledge or perspective.

The **Realpolitik** *of evidence*

However dubious or even cynical one might be about modern politics, the politics of 'spin' or politicians themselves, it is nevertheless the case that beneath the clever rhetoric there is often a hardnosed political realism at work. This *Realpolitik* is primarily based on practical considerations when it comes to influencing public opinion, diplomacy and evaluating policy measures. In this sense, it is therefore unsurprising that we should discover a significant concluding verdict on the veracity of evidence-based practice in the political arena of government. What is perhaps more unusual is that we might trace this political realism in the UK context to a close inspection of a set of minutes, reports and oral evidence from a House of Commons Science and Technology Select Committee, reported on 26 October 2006. This Select Committee, chaired by Phil Willis MP (Liberal Democrat), was tasked with inquiring into the government's handling of 'scientific advice, risk and evidence in policy making'. Its findings and recommendations regarding evidence-based policy and practice are most revealing for the central arguments we pursue in this book. Before expounding on the main findings and recommendations of the

Select Committee, some background information will be helpful to the reader.

Reforming and modernizing the machinery of government was a central feature of the Blair administrations of 1997 and 2001. Part of this modernization and reform was a commitment to evidence-based policy. The *Modernising government* white paper (Cabinet Office 1999a), for instance, stated that government policy must be evidence-based, properly evaluated and grounded on best practice. A report from the Cabinet Office Strategic Policy Making Team, *Professional policy making for the twenty-first century* (Cabinet Office 1999b), suggested that 'policy making must be soundly based on evidence of "what works"' and that 'government departments must improve their capacity to make use of evidence'. However, and contrary to this, the House of Commons Science and Technology Select Committee Report (2006: 3), on the government's handling of scientific advice, risk and evidence, summarized that, 'in considering evidence based policy, we conclude that the Government *should not overplay this mantra*, but should acknowledge more openly the many drivers of policy making, as well as any gaps in the relevant research base' (emphasis added). The Committee made explicit the links between the evidence-based agenda and the controversial 'what works' movement, stating that the former is 'not a new concept, [it] has its roots in Government's commitment to "what works" over ideologically driven policy, and in the Modernising Government agenda' (*ibid.*: 11). The Select Committee's report recommended that:

> Government needed to conduct evaluation 'not just to show "what works" but also why policies work (or not), and what we understand of current phenomena and likely future trends in shaping policies and outcomes'. This echoes comments made by Norman Glass: '"What works" is important, but "how it works" … is equally, if not more, important'.
> (House of Commons Science and Technology Select Committee 2006: 58, 118)

In its concluding recommendation, the Select Committee (2006: 64, 124) said: 'We have argued that the phrase "evidence based policy" is *misleading* and that the Government should therefore desist from seeking to claim that all its policies are evidence based' (emphasis added). Let us look in more detail at the recommendations and written and oral contributions made to the Select Committee as a way of evaluating the current status of evidence-based practice within the all-important political dimension.[25]

A former Treasury civil servant, Norman Glass (director of the National Centre for Social Research) was especially critical of the Treasury's approach to evidence-based policy evaluation, commenting that 'Systematic evaluation of policies (even where it exists and the Treasury itself is a notable non-practitioner) remains, in many cases, a procedure for bayoneting the dead' (House of Commons Science and Technology Select Committee 2006: 59, 118). William Solesbury (director of the ESRC's Centre for Evidence Policy and Practice) suggested that a National Audit Office-style body should be established to assess the evidence basis of policy, but the Secretary of State for Trade and Industry, Rt Hon. Alistair Darling (currently Chancellor of the Exchequer under the Brown government), was skeptical. He reported 'doubts as to whether or not it is possible to get somebody who was so distant, so impartial', noting that different people 'will *look at the same evidence and come to different conclusions*' (emphasis added) about whether it is reflected by the policy (*ibid.*: 60, 120). The Select Committee shared his skepticism (*ibid.*: 60, 120). Later, in response to questioning about evidence that speed cameras reduce accidents and save lives, the Secretary of State admitted that evidence-based policy is incompatible with government:

> I think, in general, evidence ought to be published, and if you look at speed camera stuff I can think of at least two major studies that were published and are there. I can tell you, there are 57 different views on what we ought to do with it, because people look at evidence, and of course most people are adept at interpreting evidence in a way that suits their purpose.
>   (Science and Technology: Evidence Ev 71, 5 July 2006, Q1316)[26]

Then, Secretary of State Darling rather throws the baby out with the bathwater, admitting that in spite of the evidence, 'there comes a time when you say, "You use your judgment." There could be other things where there is evidence that something works, and, for perfectly good policy reasons, we say it is not the thing we want to do' (Ev.72, Q1322). Here, Darling is emphasizing that what counts is not the evidence, but expert judgement as an act of interpretation that is made on the basis of some sort of evidence, and moreover that even in the face of the evidence, it is a matter of necessity that judgements are made that run contrary to it. What is most striking about this admission is that, after a decade or more of heavy government investment into an evidence-based infrastructure and policy formation, the Secretary of State is effectively cutting the movement loose. Both the Select Committee and Darling question whether an evidence-based policy was, in fact, ever feasible. The summary recommendation by the Select Committee stated: 'We agree that ministerial decisions need to take into account factors other than evidence, but this is not reflected in the Government's oft-repeated assertion that it is committed to pursuing an evidence *based* approach to policy making'. And it followed up with: 'It would be more honest and accurate to acknowledge the fact that while evidence plays a role in informing policy, decisions are ultimately based on a number of factors – including political expediency' (House of Commons Science and Technology Select Committee 2007, Recommendation 35). This, of course, begs the question that if political expediency as the basis for professional decision-making is good enough for policy implementers, then surely it should be acknowledged as being good enough for frontline social workers? William Solesbury expanded upon the Secretary of State's oral evidence as follows:

> I think the concept that policy should be based on evidence is something that I would rail against quite fiercely. It implies first of all that it is the sole thing that you should consider. Secondly, it implies the metaphor 'base' and

implies a kind of solidity, which … is often not there, certainly in the social sciences although I think to a great degree … not always in the natural and biological sciences.

> (House of Commons Science and Technology Select Committee
> 2007: 45, 85)

We finish this section with Solesbury's admissions to the Select Committee that '"Evidence informed policy and practice" is nearer the reality' (*ibid.*) and that the term 'evidence-based' was imposed on his research centre by the ESRC (*ibid.*). Glass agreed, saying 'I do not like the phrase "evidence based" – it is not the way policy gets made' and that, in deferring to natural scientists, he wished he had 'the chance to do experiments in the way they do experiments' (*ibid.*). Judy Nixon, from Sheffield Hallam University, argued that evidence-based practice had been used to distort the justification of Anti-Social Behaviour Orders (ASBOs) and that her research had encountered 'examples of more tenuous relationships between policies and the evidence on which they were purported to be based than is suggested by the phrase "evidence-based practice"' (House of Commons Science and Technology Select Committee 2007: 46, 87).

Conclusion

In this chapter, we have laid out the foundations for an alternative and, we feel, persuasive way of understanding evidence-based social work as an actor network. Our analysis demonstrates how actor network theory offers a strategy to track and map the formalization of evidence-based practice in its various articulations in social work. By using the UK case context and anchoring our theoretical and methodological premises in actor network theory, we have endeavoured to show how networked actors enrol other actors – human or non-human – through translations, i.e., aligning their interests through arguments, negotiations and detours, in a strategic effort to become indispensable or normative. The analysis has revealed how alliances, convergences and connections occur that allow the evidence network to acquire power through the number, extensiveness and stability of the connections routed through them. Certain actors and institutions are seen to enlist texts, artefacts, research methods, policy initiatives and processes as 'enrolled' or 'allied' players. The strategizing that takes places within the evidence network consists of a set of processes that generate accommodation between loosely aligned epistemological and political values that need to be formalized, but, at the same time, are sources of tension and dispute. Since a fundamental problem of the evidence-based strategist is to ensure the legitimacy of their particular worldview, the process of strategy formation will necessarily be an exercise of demonstration, often couched in language like 'what works' or 'scientific credentials'. We have seen how network stabilizations between a set of actors or institutions aim increasingly at stability and predictability, through the mantra of evidence-based social work, and ultimately push for uniformity, accountability and the standardization of frontline practice. A key lesson we have learnt from the above analysis is that 'To adopt an innovation is to adapt it' (Akrich *et al.* 2002b: 12) – such is the formula which best explains the diffusion of evidence-based practice. In this respect, we have seen that as part of the enrolment process, those championing evidence-based practice, such as SCIE, are also pressed to incrementally adjust the conception of the method to fit the context. Thus implicit in the SCIE strategy has been the adaptation of a 'soft' and 'hard' approach to evidence-based social work as a way of responding flexibly to different audiences and critics, as well as positioning itself in relation to major stakeholders across time. Generally, this is done in order to establish a satisfying compromise between its characteristics, criticism and the myriad demands of users such as governments, policy-makers, managers, researchers and frontline practitioners. In the next chapter, we narrow the lens of our actor network analysis to focus on the way this has been undertaken in various implementation strategies that have been developed in relation to evidence-based social work.

Notes

1   Given the huge proliferation of evidence-based initiatives in the UK over the past decade (conferences, groups, organizations, centres, institutes and networks), it would be impossible to discuss and evaluate each and every one. Therefore, we have concentrated chronologically on those that have had a significant impact on shaping the evidence-based agenda in social work and identified some of the key markers and actors in the network development of evidence-based practice in the UK.

2   Callon (1986) outlines the process of translation as having four 'moments'. The first, which he calls *problematisation* or 'how to become indispensable', is the one in which key actors define the nature of the problem and the roles of other actors to fit the solution proposed. The second moment, *interessement* or 'how allies are locked in place', is a series of processes which attempt to impose the identities defined in the problematization on the other actors. The third moment, *enrolment* or how to define and coordinate the roles that will then follow, leads to the establishment of a stable network of alliances. For enrolment to be successful requires others to yield (Singleton and Michael 1993). Finally, *mobilisation* or 'are the spokespersons representative?' occurs as the proposed solution gains wider acceptance and an even larger network of absent entities is created (Grint and Woolgar 1997) through some actors taking on the role as spokespersons for others.

3   In various articles Ian Sanderson has undertaken a critique of the political rationality of 'what works'. He emphasizes the role of evidence in policy-making as being indicative of a 'technocratic politics' underpinned by an instrumental rationality which erodes the normative basis of policy-making and undermines the capacity for 'appropriate' practice. Sanderson (2002: 61) argues that the current emphasis on evidence-based practice needs to be understood in the context of recent trends in governance processes and the development by New Labour of performance management for public services. Also see Paul Scourfield's article in *Critical Social Policy*, 2006.

4   http://cat.inist.fr/?aModele=afficheN&cpsidt=16960172

5   The Campbell Collaboration was officially founded in Pennsylvania in 2000.

6   http://www.campbellcollaboration.org/papers/4_progress.pdf

7   http://www.ucl.ac.uk/spp/download/publications/SPP-FIN.pdf

8   http://www.ucl.ac.uk/spp/download/publications/SPP-FIN.pdf

9   MacKenzie's (1996) analysis of the role of the self-fulfilling prophecy in technological development is relevant here. In a similar way to the diffusion model discussed in Chapter 4, he shows that beliefs that the speed of computers would continue to increase

at a regular rate provided goals for computer companies, which in turn created the computers conforming to expectations.

10 CEBSS Newsletters and reports spanning 1999–2004 have been archived by the *Research in Practice* group and are available at http://www.ripfa.org.uk/aboutus/ archive/index.asp?TOPcatID=6

11 NICE provides authoritative and prescriptive advice on the effectiveness of interventions to improve health and reduce health inequalities and on treatments and the best clinical practice.

12 See Chapter 6 for a brief discussion of the activities of Research in Practice and the UK university social work department grouping Making Research Count.

13 http://www.scie.org.uk/publications/knowledgereviews/kr12.asp

14 The passage to network centrality and expert mastery for SCIE is not an easy one. Credibility and legitimation for SCIE initially occur as 'peripheral participation', which Lave and Wenger (1991) view as an enculturation process. As part of this process, SCIE, as a newcomer, needed to gain recognition by gradually becoming part of a 'community of practice' in social work, thereby acquiring confirmation and approval as a grouping of evidence-based experts. SCIE's reconnaissance trips, user involvement and stakeholder participation agenda did much to ease the passage in this respect.

15 The famous US social work reformer and philanthropist Jane Addams was awarded a Barnett House Fellowship in the early twentieth century.

16 http://www.spsw.ox.ac.uk/fileadmin/static/cebi/

17 The 'three-strikes and you're out' mentality originated in the USA. It was a 'what works' policy initiative in criminal sentencing whereby state courts were required to hand out mandatory periods of incarceration to criminals who had been convicted of three offences, and a policy that California governor Arnold Schwarzenegger has been particularly keen to enforce.

18 The Platt Review also attacked the *British Journal of Social Work* for being 'too theoretical' and postmodern in orientation and engaged in an unsubstantiated and exaggerated set of criticisms against its editorial policy. The editors, Eric Blyth and Helen Masson, responded with a fairly tame but defensive retort.

19 See Board meeting minutes (http://www.scie.org.uk/publications/corporate/minutes-jul07.pdf).

20 http://www.scie.org.uk/about/index.asp

21 http://www.scie.org.uk/news/mediareleases/2008/071008.asp. The National Skills Academy aims to improve productivity and tackle skills shortages across the UK. They include skills academies in the financial services, construction, manufacturing, food and drink manufacturing, nuclear and process industries *and* social care.

22 The website for the Evidence Network is housed at Kings College, University of London, and acts as an information broker and gateway for evidence-based policy and practice (http://www.kcl.ac.uk/schools/sspp/interdisciplinary/evidence).

23 http://www.kcl.ac.uk/content/1/c6/03/20/26/evidencepolicyflyer2008.pdf and http://www.policypress.org.uk/journals/evidence_policy/

24 http://eppi.ioe.ac.uk/cms/

25 http://www.publications.parliament.uk/pa/cm200506/cmselect/cmsctech/900/6052401.htm

26 http://www.publications.parliament.uk/pa/cm200506/cmselect/cmsctech/900/900-ii.pdf

6   Making evidence a reality?

In Chapter 5, we saw how the success of evidence-based social work is, to a large extent, dependent on enrolling participants by locking them into a solid chain of translations. These translations involve performative as well as structural components, whereby the champions of evidence-based social work are engaged in intense activities of enrolling, enlisting and convincing potential converts. The way in which the network gets formed depends on the mobility of actors and organizations and their ability to shift between roles and relations. It was illustrated how actor network theory offers a strategy to track and map evidence-based practice (EBP) in its various expressions, through the networks it influences as well as through its controversial and more silent articulations.[1] This chapter, in its formulation of implementation factors for evidence-based social work, persists with the actor network framework and is anchored in its theoretical and methodological articulation. Towards the end of the chapter, we construct a way of thinking about the implementation of evidence-based practice in social work in strategic terms and one that recognizes organizational, professional and intervention complexities as dynamic and fluid (Neyland 2006).

In Chapter 5, we demonstrated how, through the networks of key actors, organizations and policies, and an emergent research infrastructure, evidence-based practice has become part of a global social work discourse. This discourse is generated through a form of mobilization, and its inherent presence through what is a process of implementation can be found through these. It is this very important and decisive issue of implementation that we turn to in this chapter. Towards the end of the chapter, we contrast the implementation strategy for evidence-based social work with a knowledge transfer model. Crucially with these considerations, the relation between 'universally applicable' evidence-based knowledge and local, indigenous professional knowledge comes to the fore. That is, the problem of 'the general and the particular', whereby the production of general principles to cover a wide array of activities attempts to be enacted in particular circumstances. We saw in Chapter 4 how actor network analyses have focused on the distinction between universally applicable 'scientific' knowledge and 'local' knowledge. This opposition has mobilized considerable research advancing our understanding of what happens when science leaves the laboratory and enters the world of application in other 'localities' (Latour 1987; Law and Hassard 1999; Murdoch 1998).

We have witnessed how, in actor network terms, evidence-based practice needs to translate (Callon 1986) into social work in a form where it can be adopted. As part of a complex process, this may mean choosing some elements of the innovation to keep in and other elements to leave out. Negotiation, diplomacy and the mobilization of power relations are important features that are often overlooked in implementation literature on evidence-based practice. Most implementation research lacks a sense of the political interaction of stakeholders that is fundamental to understanding the public sector. Agrawal (2005) stresses the central role of power in the negotiation of knowledge networks and the subject formation of professional expert identity. To be effective, scientists and policy advocates must negotiate knowledge with often powerful subjects and objects of other network segments. For the champions of evidence-based social work, this has meant making a number of critical compromises and deals based on their assessment of the receptivity of social work professionals and managers, as well as judgements about the feasibility of certain methodologies and practices over others. In a very important way, this occurred with the deliberate softening of the more rigid scientific parameters of the medical model for evidence-based practice to make it more palatable for its messier social dimensions. In this respect, in the previous chapter we noticed how the Campbell Collaboration and SCIE were central translation agencies in adjusting the appropriation of evidence-based practice from their medical allies in the Cochrane Collaboration and the National Institute for Clinical Excellence (NICE). An advocacy coalition is formed by setting policy agendas and framing complementary strategies, e.g., information management and casework management systems, between these different knowledge network segments. This example of network translations across different public sector segments concerned with evidence-based implementation illustrates the importance of strategic alliances as a feature of a socio-political dimension. Researchers who concentrate solely on the technological innovations of evidence-based practice as the driving force are likely to produce an imbalanced account of the implementation issues. It is our contention that evidence-based social work is, by its very nature, a socio-technical innovation. Thus we wish to illustrate how the process of implementation is also both a social and technical exercise that is strategically grounded. Research into the implementation and operation of evidence-based social work needs to take into account this heterogeneity and find a way to give due regard to both the social and technical aspects of its elaboration. With the technical dimension, there are important considerations about computer-based systems, information management systems, web-development sites, electronic record systems, software data and operating systems, as well as electronic or 'hard-copy' documentation, such as guidelines and procedural manuals. The implementation of evidence-based practice, as a way of upgrading existing systems, should be viewed in terms of a technological innovation. At a formal level, the social dimension that relates to the implementation of evidence-based practice is constructed through policy and best practice guidelines that are expected to redirect professional actions and reshape interventions in a certain way, as prescribed by its advocates. At an informal level, however, there are a diverse set of social factors ranging from the perceived threat of evidence-based practice on professional values and identity to a lack of local knowledge, resources and expertise in being able to implement the innovation. Schematically, the implementation literature points to the significance of informal dimensions in the uptake of research for practice, such that local, indigenous knowledge networks are, within their local social work domains, dominant and therefore often capable of resisting the socio-technological incursions of evidence-based practice.

In this chapter, we examine both the formal and informal aspects of the social-technical dimension that impact on barriers in the implementation of evidence-based practice for social work. We reveal that the fate of the evidence-based practice project in social work depends on the various moves taken by different stakeholder parties and how they handle researcher and frontline practitioner resistance. This is a tricky and delicate process which implementation research tends to overlook. Effectively, every handling of the evidence-based practice project by different stakeholders could present either a positive modality – that strengthens it and pushes it forward on its track – or a negative modality – that weakens its initial form and drags it into a different direction. For some writers on implementation in social work, e.g., Mullen and Bacon (2003), only minimal expertise is required to ensure that some form of mobilization is triggered by evidence-based practice – expertise that should, in fact, be generated by the evidence-based methodology itself and the systems built around it. Thus professional learning is a critical ingredient in the uptake of evidence-based practice for frontline practitioners. However, as we shall see, while advocates of evidence-based practice encourage social workers to reorient their interventions, they give few examples of what this actually entails in the day-to-day work of frontline practice. Indeed, we demonstrate that a good proportion of the implementation literature in evidence-based social work rests on assumptions that policy recommendations, knowledge reviews and best practice guidelines are shared *a priori* among researchers, policy advisors, managers, practitioners and implementers. We show how implementation recommendations often contain only vague guidance for practice, with advocates of evidence-based social work working under incomplete or simply idiosyncratic understandings of what evidence-based policy means for frontline practice. Moreover, the implementation literature is overly concerned with changing individual practitioner behaviour. The very straightforward matter of how a social work practitioner faced with a large and varied caseload – including domestic violence, drug dependency and substance misuse, youth offending and street crime, emotionally disturbed children, women's mental health, legislation involving looked-after children and child development issues – keeps up-to-date with evidence in each of these fields is simply ignored. Given the complex and multi-faceted situations in which social workers find themselves, it is difficult to conceive how any frontline practitioner could keep up with research findings across so many different fields. The daily pressure of case management methods, whereby social workers are expected to see more clients, makes it extremely difficult for practitioners to find the time to read research literature, even if they were inclined to do so. The problems associated with the lack of fit between, for example, best practice guidelines for evidence-based social work and the realities of frontline practice are also taken up in a focused way in the concluding chapter.

Barriers to implementation

Implementation theory is fairly familiar to researchers and policy-makers within the evidence-based field, since it is concerned with demonstrating how the implementation of policy and intervention strategies either succeed or fail and how best to ensure that they are not subverted. It is empirical, behavioural and linear in orientation. Over the past ten years, there has been a huge research investment in these kinds of studies in social policy and social work.[2] This first part of the chapter focuses on this straightforward approach to issues surrounding the implementation of evidence-based practice in social work. To give the flavour of the centrality of implementation theory in social work, Proctor and Rosen (2008: 258) typically define 'implementation studies' as 'examining the acceptability of evidence-based interventions, the feasibility and likelihood of their sustained use, and the decision-support procedures that can help practitioners apply probabilistically based, empirically supported treatments to the individual case in real-world practice'. More sophisticatedly within this genre, Hill (2003: 269) observes that 'Formally, implementation resources are defined as individuals or organizations that can help implementing units learn about policy, best practices for doing policy, or professional reforms meant to change the character of services delivered to clients'. In previous chapters, we showed that developing a professional culture within social work that is supportive of improving research for practice requires both the generation and use or application of evidence. As we shall see, this is no small task and presents significant hurdles for implementation strategists. Prospective identification of efficient strategies and barriers to change is necessary to achieve a better adaptation of intervention to improve 'best practice'. We now examine the factors that inhibit and facilitate knowledge translation of research evidence by social workers (Webb 2002) and focus on how the successful implementation of research into practice is likely to be a function of both macro and micro factors. This depends on the interplay of four core elements that constitute the interwoven implementation factors: (i) the knowledge transfer systems for evidence; (ii) the level, nature and systematicity of the evidence; (iii) the context or environment into which the research is to be disseminated; and (iv) the method, or way in which, the process is facilitated. The factors inhibiting knowledge translation and the implementation of evidence-based policy are likely to be complex and entrenched. The issues inhibiting evidence-based social work include a range of macro and micro dimensions.

For the purposes of this discussion, 'implementation' is normatively defined as a specified set of activities designed to put into practice an activity or program of known dimensions. For social work, the effective implementation of evidence-based practice is increasingly regarded as a component that is as important as the intervention itself, with 'implementation for impact' as the goal (Sheldon 2001). The objective of implementing evidence-based practice in social work is to create reliable, satisfactory outcomes for service users through interventions based on valid research findings. To accomplish this, high-fidelity professional decision-making must be developed, supported and sustained (Gira *et al*. 2004). In medical parlance, this is referred to as 'treatment fidelity'. In intervention fields, such as social work and medicine, 'treatment fidelity' is defined as the strategies that monitor and enhance the accuracy and consistency of an intervention to ensure that it is implemented as planned and that each component is delivered in a comparable manner to all service users over time. This is essential if valid and reliable research on intervention effectiveness is to be done in a way that is transferable across contexts – such that programs from the USA, for example, might be applied in Norway and Sweden, as was the case with multi-systemic therapy (MST), discussed in Chapter 4. Without treatment fidelity, meaningful comparisons cannot be made.

There are considerable barriers to implementing evidence-based social work, some of which have received little systematic research attention. Implementing evidence-based practice in social work is fragmented and variable. Barriers ranging from negative practitioner attitudes to administrative steering failure constitute the breadth of problems. Some problems of implementation derive from the fact that evidence-based practice has offered simplistic solutions: if researchers would produce practice-relevant, evidence-based models, then practitioners would find, adopt and use them (Barber, in White 2008; Mullen and Bacon 2004). Barratt (2003: 146) found that few organizations or practitioners held common views regarding the nature of evidence and that little consensus existed on how such research evidence could be effectively utilized. In addition, there was little clarity about the types of mechanisms needed to promote and sustain an evidence-based culture. She found considerable consensus on the need for organizations to share a common understanding of what constitutes 'best research evidence'.

Hodson (2003) found that a combination of micro and macro approaches was more likely to achieve lasting change in developing a research-evidence culture. Micro approaches refer to intervention resources and to altering the attitudes, ways of working and behaviours of individual practitioners, while macro approaches relate to the top-down strategy of redesigning key systems, such as the system for the dissemination of evidence.

Macro factors

Cultural factors

Cultural factors influence uptake and dissemination efforts. Producers of evidence guidelines (typically, academic researchers) and users of research evidence (usually policy-makers and practitioners) often have different values, goals and perspectives that are shaped by professional cultures. Cultural differences, such as professional values, mould the key questions that researchers and practitioners use to make decisions. Indeed, the working culture of social work is a somewhat closed practice – that is, one in which frontline practitioners do not expect their more detailed judgements and decisions to be warranted by rigorous and systematically collected evidence.

Practitioners report that evidence-based guidelines cannot be used for decision-making when the key questions addressed do not correspond to real questions. Practitioners making decisions sometimes do not understand that some questions are not researchable, while researchers sometimes answer questions other than those posed by decision-makers. These tensions need to be examined to delineate a sound balance for evidence-based practice integration in different environments (Mullen, Bellamy *et al.* 2005).

Barratt (2003: 148) highlights the problem of risk-aversive and blame culture mentalities in social work agencies as a deterrent to using evidence-based practice (see also Webb 2006). She mentions that:

> Most respondents supported a view that the existence of 'blame cultures' prevented both practitioners and planners being experimental when applying research to practice. The fear of 'getting it wrong' encouraged agencies and staff to remain within the boundaries of existing practice and assumptions – regardless of the potential for perpetuating ineffective practice.

The issue of deprofessionalization – and loss of professional autonomy – looms large in the minds of many critics of evidence-based social work. This may be because social workers have seen how evidence-based medicine has increasingly deskilled and deprofessionalized medical and healthcare practitioners. Lucas (2008: 92) reports as follows on the professional healthcare culture emerging around NICE:

> Although it is said that 'NICE guidance does not replace the knowledge and skills of individual health professionals who treat patients', once national guidance has been issued by NICE, it replaces local recommendations and promotes equal access for patients across the country; when NICE has not issued guidance on an 'interventional procedure', 'health professionals are expected' to 'seek approval from their NHS trust's clinical governance committee and ensure that patients' [sic] have given informed consent before carrying it out …. I know General Practitioners who feed clinical measurements into a computer model to decide whether they are 'allowed' to treat an elevated cholesterol level. Whether this is a rule of the practice in which they work, or is a way of demonstrating that they have followed NICE guidelines (and NICE guidelines can be and are referred to in General Medical Council cases into fitness to practice), *they appear to be acting as if these guidelines are rules, and that they are high-level technicians rather than fully fledged professionals* (emphasis added).

These findings from NICE are relevant to social work in that the prescribed, standardized use of a rigid, quantitative, positivistic approach is evolving into a situation whereby evidence-based health science is widely promoted as *the truth* (Murray *et al.* 2008). The accusation that evidence-based practice deprofessionalizes social work is made on the basis of it being a reductionist approach primarily intended as a cost-saving and management regulation exercise, while based on a mechanistic view of quality interventions through streamlining what is traditionally considered to be professional judgement. We have seen in Chapter 2 how evidence-based practice has a rigid hierarchy of what counts as evidence, and how this has been endorsed by research institutions, journal editors and agencies – like SCIE – that serve to reproduce the exclusion of certain forms of professional practice and knowledge production (Barber, in White 2008). Such narrow conceptions of evidence-based practice lead to claims that it is a regime which endorses only a narrow view of science, which privileges economic modes of governance and efficiency.

Strategic factors

Strategic factors relate to efforts to resolve the lack of utilization of evidence-based research in social work and the systems put in place to ensure knowledge translation. If guidelines were developed based on systematic reviews of evidence-based research, changes in decisions would not occur until systems were in place to advise service providers and support the implementation of new guidelines. At a strategic level, the development of knowledge translation systems offers important drivers to implement evidence-based practice. We have seen how knowledge translation offers a structured process for the generation, storage, distribution and application of research evidence in stakeholder organizations. Evidence-based guidelines and protocols form an important element of this strategic infrastructure (Webb 2008). Greenhalgh (2001) argues that these are increasingly used to achieve several objectives, including making standards explicit and accessible, honing professional decision-making and improving cost-effectiveness.

Environmental factors

Where the research is placed is a crucial factor influencing the use of research evidence. The research will focus on significant organizational and environmental factors. Several studies have documented the barriers to the implementation of research findings at the individual practice level, particularly in the field of healthcare (see Bero *et al*. 1998). However, less is known about the experiences of organizations adopting evidence-based practice. In the UK, barriers identified by Hampshire Social Services (1999) included the organizational culture, practice and educational environment. These barriers are representative of environmental challenges (Mullen *et al*. 2008).

Micro factors

Dissemination of research evidence

The focus here is on the effectiveness of various dissemination and micro-implementation strategies in the field. We saw in Chapter 5 how, in the UK,

SCIE has become a major driver in the dissemination of certain types of research evidence. We also noted that the development of empirically supported research runs parallel to the publication of practice guidelines, or what SCIE calls 'best practice guidelines', which attempt to capture a profession's consensus on its area of expertise and to suggest the preferred way to perform a particular intervention. Typically in the UK, the Research in Practice (RIP) group produces information about (i) how to use research evidence in service planning and selection, and (ii) how to gather research evidence to monitor and evaluate practice service. The recently published *Think research: using research evidence to inform service development for vulnerable groups* (2008) is indicative of the type of information produced. It is described as a 'user-friendly tool to assist commissioners and service providers to select and monitor evidence-informed services for vulnerable children and adults with additional needs'.[3]

In US healthcare, practice guidelines are described by the Institute of Medicine as 'systematically developed statements to assist practitioner and patient decisions about appropriate health care for specific clinical circumstances' (Field and Lohr 1990: 38). Howard and Jensen (1999: 283) summarize the situation as follows:

> Guidelines for clinical practice have proliferated in recent years. Numerous studies indicate that guidelines can increase empirically based practice and improve clients' outcomes. Guidelines for social work practice would also promote more informed client decision making, improve clinical training in schools of social work, encourage more cost-effective and accountable practice, and help codify current knowledge in controversial practice areas.

Rosen and Proctor (2003: 18) were the first to provide a book-length treatment of practice guidelines in social work, where such guidelines were defined as 'a set of systematically compiled and organized statements of empirically tested knowledge and procedures to help practitioners select and implement interventions that are the most effective for attaining desired outcomes'. They describe the components of such guidelines as comprising four areas: the targets of intervention, the array of possible interventions, the criteria used to choose among the alternative interventions for particular clients and situations, and the gaps or uncertainties of application.

Wambach *et al.* (1999) are skeptical about the value of practice guidelines in social work. They raised concerns about the implementation potential of these tools, claiming that they lack specificity and do not reduce uncertainty or assist social workers in their day-to-day activities. They provide an example from the American Psychiatric Association (1995) guidelines for interventions with people with substance use disorders. The guidelines indicate that social workers should use 'cognitive behavioral therapies, behavioral therapies, psychodynamic/ interpersonal therapies, group and family therapies, and participation' (Wambach *et al.* 1999: 323). This wish list is vague, unrealistic and unattainable for most local interventions. They also claim that practice guidelines are limited 'because the decision to adopt a particular practice guideline is more likely to occur on an agency level, rather than focused on individual practitioners' (*ibid.*). More importantly, they ask how, if social work students come to expect a step-by-step approach to practice decisions, would 'they learn to develop critical thinking skills as practitioners?' (Wambach *et al.* 1999: 324). Lastly, they contend that 'unless guideline production methodology can be adjusted to value input characterized as *practice wisdom*, it seems doubtful that the practice community will accept and use such guidelines' (*ibid.*: 328).

Despite the concerted efforts to instil a culture of guideline adherence – including those by organizations like SCIE (Mullen and Bacon 2004) – current research indicates that these guidelines are not widely used in routine social work practice. Practical concerns regarding the dissemination of guidelines suggest that the social work research database is insufficient to support broad-based guideline development. Kirk (1999: 309) contended that 'guidelines are only as good as the knowledge base' and that 'the knowledge base for social work practice is thin'. Steketee (1999: 344) raised a related concern, asserting that 'until a sufficient number of such [large studies of diverse clients with similar problems] ... has been reported in a given problem area, it is unreasonable to formulate clinical guidelines that are truly empirically supported'.

A cautionary warning for agencies like SCIE is that the evidence from medicine and allied health professions shows that certain types of research dissemination have little impact on the adoption of evidence-based guidelines (Merritt *et al.* 1999; Woolf *et al.* 1996, 1999). This research shows that individual clinical autonomy inevitably takes precedence over the prescriptive aspect of the 'cookbook' guidelines. Perhaps with this in mind, Julie Jones, chief executive of SCIE, commented that 'We are moving away from printed documents and guides because we've learned we have to target our work much more. We can't just publish something and hope people look at it, we have to make sure it's relevant and also be very aware of future policy guidance' (*Community Care*, 22 August 2007). Timmermans (2008) summarizes the recent research findings on the adoption of clinical guidelines in medicine. He suggests that:

> If we evaluate how clinical guidelines render actual behavior uniform in the way intended by their designers, these instruments have a relatively low rate of return. The general suspicion is that 'guidelines may do little to change practice behavior' (Woolf *et al.* 1999). Although inconclusive at best, most of the available research confirms this hypothesis. First, there seems to be little awareness of guidelines. A survey of 100 New Zealand general practitioners after the release of a guideline on the management of hypertension showed that only 40% had read the guideline (Arroll *et al.* 1995). Researchers in Seattle surveyed 300 pediatricians about their knowledge and impression of four well-publicized pediatric practice guidelines (Christakis and Rivara 1998). The awareness of the guidelines varied from only 15 to 66%, and the pediatricians dismissed the guidelines as too 'cookbook,' time-consuming, and cumbersome. Self-reported change due to the guidelines varied from 19 to 36%.
>
> (Timmermans 2008: 494)

According to Timmermans (2008: 494), in reporting a number of empirical case studies, 'even if practice guidelines are known, they rarely change the behavior of professionals'. Similarly, Freemantle *et al.* (2001) reviewed eleven experiments that evaluated the effectiveness of printed educational materials in changing physician behaviour. As cited in Gira *et al.*'s (2004: 69) review of meta-analyses of these, ten studies were randomized controlled trials (RCTs) and one study used interrupted time-series analyses. The studies included interventions comparing (i) printed educational materials versus a non-intervention control, and (ii) printed educational materials plus implementation strategies versus printed educational materials alone. Results were reported as percentages of relative improvement and ranged only from 16 to 24 per cent. None of the results of these studies using educational materials alone to influence physician behaviour was statistically significant. Kirk (1999: 305) is skeptical about whether practitioners would read best practice guidelines if they 'generally do not subscribe to academic journals or read research articles'. He claims that many guidelines have little use to practitioners because of the equivocal or global nature of their recommendations and their failure to provide the 'practitioner struggling at a particular moment and setting with a particular patient and limited resources' with 'definitive advice' (Kirk 1999: 306).

Guideline adoption is not a systematic process involving the majority of professional social workers. When they are adopted, at best, the guidelines reflect routine practice and are not the basis of the formal proof of efficacy. That is, they do not produce a radical change in behaviour, but their effect is likely to result in a more nuanced, discretionary learning of when to ignore, adapt or implement guidelines. Thus it is likely that social work practitioners will view guidelines more as an option than a standardized procedure to follow. They will juggle the requirements of the guideline recommendations against the contingencies of service user care and they will negotiate with parties who have vested interests on a particular outcome.

As we shall see in the final section, there is a need for more intensive micro studies of dissemination strategies within the evidence-based agenda, moving from global analysis to highly detailed and nuanced accounts of strategic change as fragmented, hybrid flows of emergent networks. Such studies would allow us to understand how processes of improvization, purification and channelling are translated into local and national contexts, giving insights into the embedding of practice guidelines and educational material in day-to-day frontline practice contexts. Thus we might learn how guidelines are reappropriated in light of the organizational demands of frontline practice, the situational requirement and professional judgement associated with each new case. In this vein, Timmermans (2008: 152) summarizes the context of using best practice guidelines with interprofessional dynamics and organizational power, to conclude that they amount to attempts to construct professional jurisdiction over a regulated field of practice:

> What are the incentives for a profession to create clinical guidelines? Professionals are distinguished from other occupational workers by the control

they wield over the technical and formal content of their work. Sociologist Andrew Abbott (1988) used the term *jurisdiction* to refer to the link between a profession and its work. Professions have relied on credentialing, registration, and licensing mechanisms to safeguard their jurisdiction against competitors and to avoid outside evaluation of their work.

Professional education and training

Professional training includes providing specialized information, instruction or skill development in an organized way. Research shows that it is important for all personnel at all levels to receive training when a new practice, such as evidence-based practice, is implemented. Regardless of the content area, some specific training methods seem to work better than others. Some social work education programs in the UK do not include components on evidence-based practice, let alone provide appropriate coverage of implementation factors. A key question for further research is: how well does professional training equip social work practitioners to use evidence-based practice? We thus need research that will survey professional training organizations to establish the range, content and quality of evidence-based learning provision. We may define the education and training implementation theme as practitioner and educator needs for initial training and continuing education in the knowledge, skills, values and principles of evidence-based practice. Soydan (2007) asserts that social work curricula have to be reformulated and adapted to embrace the culture of evidence-based practice and emphasizes the need for course materials and tutorials that support more efficient teaching. In the USA, there is a burgeoning research literature on the professional education requirements and teaching of evidence-based practice in social work, much of which falls within a narrow scientist-as-practitioner frame of 'empirically supported interventions' (Gambrill 2007; Zlotnik 2007). Much of this literature is largely spawned through the journal *Research on Social Work Practice*. Typically, the George Warren Brown School of Social Work at Washington University has devised a new 'pedagogical paradigm' to guide educational efforts with student practitioners: 'The resolution called for instructors of all practice methods courses to teach students about the interventions that have best survived rigorous empirical testing in their respective practice areas' (Howard *et al.* 2003: 236). They suggest that one of the first questions that students should be taught as part of their evidence-based training is 'Can this direct practice or policy intervention be replicated'. They need to know 'which propositions are amenable to testing and falsification and the degree to which the evidence obtained is consistent with predictions derived from the theory' (*Ibid.*: 244). Thus it seems that for the students at the Warren Brown School of Social Work, training in social work will increasingly come to closely resemble that of a chemistry or engineering student. We are not making a cheap point here. It is very apparent that these sorts of pedagogical declarations are underpinned by a narrow hypothetico-deductive epistemology that dominates methodology teaching in the natural sciences. Indeed, Howard *et al.* (2003: 247) go on to say that social work training should be 'founded on solid scientific findings which should be distinguished from those that have not been evaluated or that are empirically unsupported'. More generally, the authors note that a curriculum incorporating evidence-based practice principles will require access to information sources, including empirical reports published in journals and books, systematic reviews, treatment manuals and practice guidelines. In an evidence-based practice curriculum, students will need to be skilled in accessing and interpreting systematic reviews, reading treatment manuals and understanding practice guidelines. Enola Proctor (2007: 587) agrees with this scientific perspective and claims that the social work 'curriculum should serve as the cornerstone for students' education for EBP'. However, she is very worried about the current state of play in US social work training courses for developing evidence-based social workers. She imagines that 'social work education shares culpability for the nation's insufficient supply of EBP-trained practitioners' (Proctor 2007: 586). It appears then that a nation-state without an ample supply of evidence-based practitioners is bereft and impoverished, with social work education shouldering some of the blame for this state of affairs. Nevertheless, she finishes on a high note in her discussion of the possible advantages for training in partnership for evidence-based social work with the announcement that 'A "win, win, win" perspective should drive these partnerships' (Proctor 2007: 591). Indeed, in the USA the enthusiasm for pedagogical reform of social work education, along evidence-based lines, shows no bounds – such that Howard *et al.* (2007: 561) call for all social work training courses to:

> ... establish a committee responsible for tracking and implementing demonstrably effective instructional innovations related to evidence-based practice; provide education courses that only promote scientifically supported practices and reward faculty who model superior pedagogical skills in relation to evidence-based practice.

They follow this with the assertion that 'Effective social workers who routinely deliver EBP interventions are, *necessarily, skilled information scientists*' (Howard *et al.* 2007: 563, emphasis added). A cynical reading of these bizarre recommendations suggests that Deleuze's 'societies of control' are alive and kicking in the social engineering efforts of certain US social work educators.

To summarize this section in terms of barriers to implementation, research has shown a lack of training in both the principles of evidence-based practice and its execution. It has been observed that there are training gaps at graduate, postgraduate and post-qualifying levels. The challenge of keeping training and continuing education up-to-date, in view of the ever-changing evidence base, is seen as a considerable barrier.[4]

There is also the important factor of social work agencies themselves providing training and staff development in evidence-based practice. In the UK, social work agencies are providing minimal staff development resources in training practitioners in evidence-based practice. Barratt (2003: 148) shows that there is a 'limited approach to continual professional development in social care. Staff development departments were not thought to take as active a role in promoting evidence based practice as they might, and it was suggested that this could inhibit the development of an evidence based culture.'

Accessibility

As the volume of research evidence expands, the scarcity of credible evidence compounds the difficulty faced by many practitioners when making decisions about which evidence to use. Concerns about gaining access to evidence relate not only to the provision of information services, but also to the individual's ability to appraise the available evidence critically and make decisions accordingly (Webb and Harlow 2003). Thus social workers may experience problems in interpreting and using research products, when they are viewed as being too complex, academic and statistical. Therefore, the presentation and management of research knowledge in frontline agencies is likely to be a significant challenge in getting research-based information into practice.

Research has shown that healthcare professionals want access to resources at the workplace, and doctors, in particular, prefer to do their own searching. Preferring individualized decision-support systems, many health professionals doubted whether a librarian could find the relevant research articles, suggesting the need for better promotion of library services in support of evidence-based practice (Lewis *et al.* 1998). While the internet provides free access to databases – such as Medline, ISTAHC, INAHTA, DARE, electronic libraries and specialized professional sites – there is often limited access to the full text of electronic papers, reviews and reports in social work agencies, which will inevitably also result in incomplete searches. A number of information management initiatives have taken place in the health, education and social care sectors to improve accessibility to evidence data.

As an example of good practice, Farrel *et al.* (1999) report on e-STABLISH, a two-year pilot project initiated in 1998 and funded by the UK's National Health Service (NHS) Executive (North West) to set up a Local Multidisciplinary Evidence Centre (LMEC) across Salford and Trafford district. The aim of e-STABLISH was to provide primary healthcare team members (PHCTs) and community staff based at twelve sites across the district with improved access to evidence-based information sources and data from their workplaces.

Time and resource factors

A barrier persistently reported from studies of social workers and clinicians across a range of professions is a perceived lack of time to adopt an evidence-based approach. In a study of four groups of health professions within two UK NHS trusts, Closs and Lewin (1998) reiterated that the lack of time for both reading and implementing research evidence remained a pervasive barrier to research utilization. Resource factors can strongly influence the success of any dissemination effort. The problem of resource constraints – including access, workspace, managerial leadership and support, and supervision and staff development programs – has been a consistently reported negative factor in barriers to implementing evidence-based practice. Little is known about how social workers collect and gather information. There are no known studies that have investigated practitioner information-gathering behaviour, the amount of information they find or the diversity of the information. Relatively little work has investigated practitioners' internet information-gathering behaviour or the amount of time they spend searching the internet. It is likely that perceived strategic environmental uncertainty affects the amount and type of information scanning that social workers engage in. If individuals are constrained by their social networks, having only a few redundant ties, then even a strong motivation to gather information may not result in a greater amount and diversity of information.

Information technology

Information systems and internet-based interactive expert systems offer great potential for accessing evidence-based knowledge on demand (Webb and Harlow 2003). They act as decision-support systems, whereby computerized applications to support evidence-based practice tend to follow a hierarchy in which systems tasks range in complexity from reference retrieval and the processing of transactions to more complex decision-support systems (Crisp 2004). Important information technology (IT) skills for implementing evidence-based practice include: knowing the information ecology; having the ability to efficiently access and search; being able to undertake information retrieving and having the capacity to store electronic information; and learning the scope and functionality of relevant databases, web search engines and meta-sites (Mullen and Bacon 2006). Current IT applications in social work can be divided into three categories: (i) *infrastructure*, such as electronic social care records (ESCRs), storage and retrieval systems, automated mechanisms for capturing data, and electronic libraries of social care literature; (ii) *performance enhancement*, such as computer-based decision-support (CDS) systems, and continuing education; and (iii) *performance evaluation*, such as demonstration and measurement of the cost, effectiveness and outcomes of different systems. All three applications can support the delivery of evidence-based social work.

Social workers with greater access to relevant and diverse information are better able to make sense of equivocal events in their environment, to notice emerging trends and problems, and to reflect on the nature of evidence. As Mark Watson (2003: 60) observes for healthcare, the internet is likely to be the most valuable information technology for evidence-based social work. In the UK, 'there have been a range of digital/electronic developments in the academic and practice settings. The main development in the social care sector has been the electronic Library for Social Care (eLSC).'[5] This electronic resource has now moved to SCIE at http://www.scie-socialcareonline.org.uk. Similarly, the group Making Research Count is a UK collaborative research dissemination initiative, which includes dissemination finds and quality research briefings.[6] Another group called Research in Practice (RIP) has a website which contains 'products' that agencies in the research-in-practice network have generated to help support or spread evidence-informed practice in their organization. This group was established 1996 at the Dartington Hall Trust, run in collaboration with the Association of Directors of Children's Services, the University of Sheffield and a network of participating agencies in the UK. They also have an 'evidence-based data bank' to provide internet-based resources. However, resources for the use and application of IT are often scarce in social work agencies. In Barratt's (2003: 146) study, 'Eighty-two per cent of respondents agreed that investment in information technology was essential to support evidence-based practice, although 20% were unsure if internet access should be made freely available to all practitioners'.

Professional decision-making

Decision-making is a complex and multi-faceted phenomenon that is necessarily subject to specific organizational environments and socio-cultural contexts (Webb 2008). The 'gold standard' expectation is that the evidence will directly inform professional decision-making. Magill (2006: 106) takes a hard line in relation to what she calls 'clinical decision making and effective interventions'. She complains that implementation strategies in social work fail precisely because they have been preoccupied with best practice guidelines and have refused to take up the crucial link between evidence and decision-making. Magill (2006) calls for explicit points of reference, or pathways that guide clinical decision-making in social work as a capacity that distinguishes the expert from the helper:

> While the merits of particular methodologies will continue to be a matter of debate, a more immediate concern is the absence of a valid and applicable framework for guiding practice decisions. Few will dispute that there must be elements of both flexibility and regimen in the treatment of psychological and social difficulties. As such, evaluation findings are intended to act as guidelines, and not precise directives.
>
> (Magill 2006: 106)

It is her contention that what remains lacking is 'an operationalized decisional strategy' (*ibid.*). Following Gambrill (1999), and endorsing a medical-clinical decision pathway model for social work, she argues that the 'Grounds for clinical decision making must move beyond intuition, gut, and theoretical preference' (*ibid.*: 107). The uncritical treatment of the evidence-based literature by Magill (2006), the appropriation of a narrow medical model, as well as the failure to address research in cognitive decision-making leave the reader feeling that a missionary zeal is at work in the article.

There is, however, a significant blind spot in Magill's (2006) argument and her treatment of clinical decision-making as the sacred cow that will cleanse social work of all non-scientific aspects of professional judgement. The blind spot is that professionals and experts do not make decisions on the basis of evidence, even when it is presented to them. Cognitive heuristics research shows conclusively that even if practitioners do act consistently, it is possible that their decisions are biased even in the face of evidence (Webb 2001). Individuals consistently fail to respect the canons of rationality assumed by the evidence-based approach. Cognitive heuristics influence decision-making to induce experts to attend to certain forms of information and to ignore others in developing professional judgements (Kahneman *et al.* 1982). Broadly speaking, a cognitive heuristic is a device that allows a decision to be made, as it were, by a rule of thumb, without full attention being paid to all available evidence. This makes for frugal, economical, but sometimes erroneous, processing of information. Thus, decision-making in social work is both enhanced and impaired by cognitive heuristics (Webb 2001).

Kahneman and Tversky (1973) showed that people fail to be influenced by base-rate evidence in reaching accurate judgements about a given situation. Nisbett and Ross (1980: 115–116), working on a proposition made by Bertrand Russell that 'popular induction depends on the emotional interest of the instances, not upon their number', argue that the effect of consensual evidence is based on subjective viewpoints rather than the sheer number of instances reported. They demonstrate that 'people are unmoved by the sorts of dry statistical data that are dear to the hearts of scientists and policy planners ... information that the scientist regards as highly pertinent and logically compelling are habitually ignored by people'. Case conference situations confirm this. When social workers provide reasons, explain decisions or conduct to other professionals or clients, they are interested in providing a justification, in putting their acts in a good light. They are also concerned to show that what they did was the right, reasonable, correct, prudent thing to do, or at least in pleading that it was permissible or excusable in some way. Recent research in heuristics undermines the insistence made by advocates of evidence-based practice as a data-driven information 'cookbook' process, whereby valid and reliable decisions are reached on the basis of empirical data or clinical guidelines (Nisbett and Ross 1980). People simply do not act or behave in this way, even when they have evidence at their disposal. The link between evidence-based practice and rational-choice decision-making is made by van de Luitgaarden (2007: 10), who notes that:

> ... aspects of social work decision making lie beyond the boundary conditions ... required to be able to validly apply analytical decision-making styles. It has been shown that people are generally not very good at making unnatural quantitative judgments about probabilities, utilities or the value that they attach to something ... as is required by statistical approaches and their decision-making capacities can deteriorate as a result of over-analysing.

However, it is our contention that biases in judgement occur as a consequence of using a heuristic to predict an outcome. Studies in this field consistently show that situational, attributional and lay inference factors bias judgements away from criteria of evidence and enhance the possibility of error. As Shelley Taylor (1981: 198) puts it, 'The past few decades have witnessed a shift away from the view of judgements as the products of rational, logical decision making marred by the occasional presence of irrational motives towards the view of the person as a heuristic user'. The various biases of human judgement in the face of evidence are often classified as either motivational or cognitive in origin (Ross 1977).

In real-life situations, and faced with clinical guidelines, practitioners will truncate the search process as soon as enough information has come to mind to form a judgement with sufficient subjective certainty. Contrary to the linear and behaviourist information process, decision-making rests on subjective experiences – of ease or difficulty of recall – that serve as a source of evidence in their own right. As Schwarz (1998: 99) showed, this subjective experience constitutes a source of information that is distinct from both the content that has been brought to mind and the information that is presented directly as evidence to the person making a judgement.

Research demonstrates that we rarely retrieve all evidence that may bear on an issue, but base our judgements on the subset of relevant information that is most accessible in memory (Bodenhausen and Wyer 1987). Kahneman and Tversky's (1973) availability heuristic holds that we form judgements of frequency, likelihood and typicality on the basis of the ease with which exemplars can be brought to mind. The wealth of cognitive science research suggests that the complex decision-making environment of social work practitioners needs to be recognized and studied in relation to evidence-based practice. Social workers are often pressured in their decisions by environmental constraints, ranging from limited resources to agency-based politics relating to the rationing of intervention outputs. For social work, it may be much more appropriate to ask what the rules are concerning decision-making, rather than what they are concerning evidence. Cognitive research suggests that memory-based reasoning has priority in expert decision-making, such that we reason from specific cases. These cases are stored in memory and accessed when the appropriate situation presents itself. However, as Stanfill and Waltz (1986) showed, in the much-cited study on memory and decision, we never simply recall a case. We modify and adapt the recollection so that it is applicable to the current situation. While acknowledging that decision-making is prone to heuristic bias, the memory-based reasoning model suggests that it nevertheless involves a very efficient and sophisticated indexing model. This model strongly confirms that decisions depend largely on past experiences articulated within a situated context and not on any evidence presented to the expert or on prescribed guideline recommendations.

It is likely that decision analysis, which has been used as a statistical technique in a number of wide-ranging areas – including water resource management, fisheries protection schemes, the disposal of radioactive waste and the handling of polluted sites, environmental hazards and nuclear medicine – will increasingly be used to regulate social work decision-making. Decision analysis or decision pathway formats are closely related to risk assessment and case management. A key strength of decision analysis is its claim to eradicate 'organizational noise' and attributes of subjective bias. It also purportedly resolves the problem of equally conflicting evidence by constructing a probabilistic ranking of decision pathway outcomes. Drawing on the mathematics of fuzzy logic, algorithms and statistical inference (discussed below), it builds attributes of individual bias and uncertainty into its probabilistic calculations of decision inputs (see Chiang 1999). It thus seeks explicitly to determine the preferences and biases of the decision-maker and the uncertainties associated with the decision. Decision analysis is intended to supplement evidence-based practice by assessing the risks and probabilities associated with social work decision processes. As Rohlin and Mileman (2000: 453) point out, 'the decision analysis approach complements that of evidence based care by enabling the best empirical evidence to be used in practice. Formal use of decision analysis will promote the rational use of existing knowledge'. Increasingly, decision software applications are created to offset bias and automate aspects of decision-making that can be expressed explicitly and maintained by database guidelines. These are all important innovations that supplement the implementation strategies and operationalization of evidence-based social work. However, it is clear that the evidence–decision interface based on this sort of cognitive science has been largely overlooked in examinations of factors influencing the uptake of research evidence.

Implementation or knowledge transfer?

So far, we have seen that there are considerable limitations associated with implementation and linear dissemination strategies for evidence-based social work. Recent research has not only questioned the reliability and validity of these implementation strategies but also raised doubts about their veracity in a number of public sector fields. The current and most fashionable parlance that is highly critical of the linear implementation strategies discussed above is referred to as a 'knowledge transfer systems' approach. This emerging concept has been defined as the exchange, synthesis and ethically sound application of knowledge within a complex system of relationships among researchers, practitioners and end users. Inasmuch as human relationships are multi-directional and interactive in nature, knowledge transfer cannot be viewed as a series of unilinear, rational actions which comprise providing, choosing and applying new knowledge from research (McWilliam 2007). In contrast to the more mechanical and behaviourist implementation strategies, the knowledge transfer model is quite distinct. As McWilliam (2007: 73) summarizes:

> KT [knowledge transfer] is not the act of transferring research-based facts to ensure clinical practice based on best evidence. A continuing education session to provide physicians with the factual evidence from a Cochrane Collaboration systematic review outlining a preferred medication protocol, for example, would not constitute KT as defined here. Nor is KT aimed at improved clinical competence and performance of individual practitioners. Thus, a continuing educational session on wound care protocol, even if refinements are premised on research studies documenting improved effectiveness, would not constitute KT as defined here. Rather, KT is an ongoing interactive human process of critically considering relevant, quality research results and findings, whether factual or tacit knowledge or humanistic understanding, blending this broader research-based knowledge with experiential knowledge

and contextual appreciation, and constructing a shared understanding and knowledge application to advance the quality of health care.

The knowledge transfer transformative strategy for linking research to practice interventions contrasts sharply with the implementation models discussed above, in that it involves professional practitioners in an on-the-job process of creating 'deeply felt interest in research findings' relevant to their everyday practice through a facilitated process of perspective transformation. As McWilliam (2007: 74) describes:

> In this KT strategy, the clinicians are provided with a brief overview of the research findings related to a specific approach to practice and several care scenarios in which this new knowledge clearly has not been applied. How these scenarios would unfold if the new knowledge were applied is also described, emphasizing provider- and client-related processes and outcomes that have been identified through the research. This process creates the 'disorienting dilemma' that Mezirow identified as foundational to contemplating the uptake and application of new knowledge.

The knowledge transfer model is organizationally and politically realistic in its ambitions. It requires that researchers, policy-makers and practitioners accept different understandings of 'evidence' than are currently widely espoused by those wishing to standardize evidence-based social work. Specifically, it endorses qualitative research findings that can inform the how-to skills and affective understanding essential to professional practice. These insights are valued additions to the factual evidence arising from the preoccupation with the narrow RCTs agenda. Effectively, the achievement of a knowledge transfer model would 'be a decentered connection of multiple practices and multiple interpretations that could be communicated between (and further disputed by) the connected strategic entities' (*ibid.*: 75) to propel the evidence-based diffusion. This onward propulsion would not necessarily aim for a fixed set of standardized goals for frontline practice but could orient toward an ongoing, disputable, connected but flexible set of principles. The knowledge transfer model, in contradistinction to linear implementation strategies, permits ambiguity and partiality that can be retained in the possibility of different elements of evidence-based social work being connected to the process, in the potential for professional expertise to redirect the process, and in the potential that the absence of fixed-end goals offer for more innovative developments.

Conclusion

We have seen that the implementation of evidence-based practice in social work is not about a single or uniform rationality, produced in a single source to have an intended effect. Drawing on the ethnographic work of Neyland (2006), we would argue that the success or failure of implementation is best understood in strategic terms as involving obligatory points of passage, from which, for example, research passes into policy and then into practice. We may ask whether implementation ever truly happens in its intended blueprint form. In this respect, an overdependence on linear modelling is extremely problematic. The implementation of evidence-based social work, its success or failure, is best understood strategically as an ongoing, contingent, achieved process.[7] For us, strategy should be seen as the linking of multiple, heterogeneous factors requiring the passage of evidence-based practice into social work to be understood through a diverse array of linked actors, networks, structures and practices. The normative expectation that surrounds the implementation of evidence-based practice in social work is that it will materialize in a more or less fixed set of locations – social work agencies or the behaviour of individual social workers – to be performed and remain durable. The emphasis is on the transportability of evidence-based practice *into* social work, based on a series of implementation moves. However, it seems to us that such fixed strategies do not work. The shift of 'movement' from implementation as an empirical leverage point to a form of behavioural practice as the articulation necessarily enables a decentering through the materialization of the agency context. Such a movement should always take account of a shifting or redistribution of the intended leverage point. This is why implementation always only ever partially happens. Therefore, we suggest that no single implementation rationality or ordering strategy is complete and, in practice, several aspects are juxtaposed together in any particular organizational or material context. Furthermore, we wish to make the general point that no implementation strategy is effective in its own right. Instead, it draws on a range of complementary practices, techniques and materials. One of the major deficits with the implementation literature for evidence-based social work is that it assumes that the passage from point A to point Z will be uncontaminated and noise free. The inflexibility of the materialized 'thing', e.g., evidence-based social work, means that the implementation strategies are often not well placed to deal with changes, ambiguity, contingency or messy instability. We believe that this is one major reason for their limited success. Indeed, it is likely that the best implementation strategy will be impure, since it will be a mix of different strategies and effects. The implementation of evidence-based social work is an embodiment of social and technical relations that do not form a coherent whole but are a set of ordering rationalities that impact on the potential for its success. The aim of implementation is to embed or achieve a stable set of organizing practices, principles and relations, often in a behavioural form. However, what gets constituted as evidence-based social work, how the assemblage is drawn together, redrawn, negotiated and resisted, is likely to be the effect of a messy and impure strategy, with much to be said for the 'reactive' liveliness, commotion and vigour of the frontline practitioners who are on the receiving end, the subject of Chapter 7.

We have seen that there are considerable barriers and challenges to implementing evidence-based practice in social work. The most obvious, and possibly the single most important factor why evidence-based social work has not obtained the leverage for adoption in countries like the UK and USA, relates to resource issues of economy and scale. Quite simply, governmental agencies have not invested sufficient funding in developing an infrastructure or in formulating a culture of evidence-based social work. Policy initiatives around research to practice in public sector organizations are always likely to be given very low priority in government-spending considerations. This is not going to change and it is unlikely that organizations like SCIE will have any significant impact on changing the behaviour of frontline practitioners. However, the situation is much more complex than this. A fuller answer to the problems of implementing evidence-based social work not only rests on economic considerations but also is determined by complex systems which develop as a result of technological specifications, professional culture, models of intervention and networked relations. Amid the political sloganeering around evidence-based practice, there is a basic tension between those who plan goals for the social care system and those who try to implement them. This tension reveals that, despite legal and administrative controls at the disposal of social work agencies, their capability to influence middle managers, who are responsible for frontline practice through innovations such as evidence-based practice, is limited by jurisdictional, institutional, functional and territorial fragmentation, and differentiation of control and responsibility in social work. This is partly because of what Nick Lee (1999) has described as the problem of 'the general and the particular', whereby the production of general principles to cover a wide array of activity cannot be enacted in particular circumstances. Thus, the lack of circulation and widespread adoption of evidence-based practice in social work needs to be understood within the more general fragmentation of networks and institutions in social work. This is due mainly to two complex factors: professional divisions that maintain some tensions and lack of communication in some instances, on the one hand, and a persistent gap between central agencies in some institutions, such as SCIE, and case managers on the other. For UK frontline practitioners, it is likely that SCIE and other organizations, like the General Social Care Council, are identified as being part of the 'centre' of regulatory social care regimes, with particular agencies and divisional teams at the 'periphery' of strategic activity. The distribution of expertise, hierarchical division and an underlying wariness by practitioners are all part of what prevents some social workers from efficiently implementing evidence-based practice. Therefore, the dominant focus on changing the behaviour of individual practitioners, through education, dissemination strategies and skilling-up to adopt an evidence-based perspective, is likely to be ineffective. The various recommendations built nationally and internationally to increase the uptake of evidence-based practice and allow it to develop its expected effects, translate in social work only into a series of weak connections of little professional impact, as comes across explicitly through the material above. The problem in the UK for evidence-based policy-makers in devising formal mechanisms of implementation occurs largely because there is a heterogeneous and largely disinterested professional practitioner workforce, local authority social services authorities and voluntary agencies, who do not act in concert, and an apparently unrepresentative organization, SCIE, supposedly representing the interests of all, which is simply far from the reality. In actor network theory terms, the evidence-based innovation often meets with an immutable social system. Apart from small pockets of activity, the overarching result is a strategic impasse.

Notes

1 By 'more silent articulations' we mean that, given the complexity of the evidence-based network and the various allegiances that it attempts to construct, it is inevitable that some connections will remain hidden and concealed even in the most thorough research process.

2 Broadly, the theoretical premise of implementation constructed by policy researchers and empirical scientists focuses on why policy does, or does not, occur as the advocates intended. In the course of developing this literature, researchers have identified more than 300 variables that might affect implementation (O'Toole 1986).

3 http://www.rip.org.uk/publications/

4 In the USA, facilitators include the increasing number of graduate programs that incorporate training in evidence-based practice, the availability of continuing education workshops and institutes that offer postgraduate training in evidence-based practice (e.g., Beck Institute for Cognitive Therapy and Research, Philadelphia, PA), and the increasing awareness on the part of social workers of the evidence base in behavioural research.

5 http://www.elsc.org.uk

6 http://www.makingresearchcount.org.uk

7 John Law (1999a: 5) describes the importance of deploying the concept of strategy to understand innovation diffusion and implementation planning as follows: strategy within a theoretical approach for interrogating the notion of power is 'the continued performance of social relations' that stabilizes through 'certain strategies for ordering these relations and their power effects'. It should be thought of as an ongoing process that treats information, strategy and connectivity to overcome distances as ongoing achievements. However, he cautions that 'If we draw on a set of discourses that have to do with strategy, then the gravitational pull of those discourses is primarily about the struggle to centre – and the struggle to centre and order from a centre. And as we know, this brings problems' (cited in Neyland 2006: 45).

7   The practitioner perspective

Consider the following fictitious scenario. In a rundown inner-city district of Oxford, UK, senior social worker Suzy Taylor has undertaken a comprehensive assessment of the McBeal family who have yet again been brought to the attention of the social work department for physically abusing their two children. Following extensive report-writing, case-file managing, risk-assessment profiling, care review and family conferences, meetings with other professionals at school, in the community, the police and the local hospital, a child protection case conference is held to make a decision on whether the two children should be received into care as 'Looked After'. Suzy has worked with the family over several years and understands the local family and community situation very well. The chair of the child protection committee refers to latest SPICE (Social Professional Institute of Clinical Evidence) 'best practice guidance', reporting that the evidence overwhelmingly suggests that the McBeal family children should become 'Looked After' and received into care. All of Suzy's professional experience, best judgement and understanding of the family situation suggest otherwise and that if she concurs with the evidence, the decision will cause real damage to the children. What does she do in the face of the evidence? In spite of the evidence-based directives and on the basis of her assessment, Suzy, using all her best skills of persuasion, makes a strong case for finding an alternative to receiving the children into care. Against the evidence, the chair of the Child Protection Committee is persuaded by Suzy's argument and 'practice wisdom', agreeing to recommend that the family receive sessions of structured family therapy and that a respite care package also be established. Three months later, Graham McBeal, aged sixteen, attacks a boy at school, causing grievous bodily harm, leading to a criminal prosecution in the local magistrate's court. Suzy Taylor is summoned to the court to provide an expert assessment. During the cross-examination, the prosecuting solicitor, referring to the SPICE 'best practice guidelines', asks Suzy why, given the evidence-based directive, Graham McBeal had not been taken into care. What does Suzy say? Has she failed to adequately represent the children's interests? She might respond by saying that after the age of fourteen, young people are considered to be fully responsible for their own actions in the same way as an adult would. However, the prosecuting solicitor would not be satisfied with this response, claiming that if Graham McBeal had become a 'Looked After' child, the probability of his committing the offence would have been greatly reduced. But would it? Promptly, but honestly, Graham interrupts the prosecuting solicitor saying that the offence was an act of revenge for a previous assault by the boy on his younger sister and that he had been planning the attack for some months. He goes on to say that even if he had been received into care, it would not have changed the outcome. Graham had not told either his family or the social worker about the premeditated revenge.

The above scenario begs important questions about the role and status of evidence in guiding professional decision-making in both social work and law. The fact of the matter with this scenario is that the evidence provided for the decision about the possibility of receiving the McBeal children into care was wholly unrelated to the grievous bodily harm incident. Moreover, there is no obvious causal or empirical connection between the physical abuse of the McBeal children by their parents and the grievous bodily harm incident by their son. And yet, the prosecuting solicitor invoked this evidence to imply that Suzy Taylor might have failed to adequately represent the McBeal children's interests. He is using evidence-based criteria to raise serious issues of legal culpability and possible professional malpractice.

We can only speculate what would happen should a legal case arise where the decision of a social worker not to follow evidence-based guidance were to be tested either in court or in the UK by the General Social Care Council under its 'code of conduct' regulations. At what point does evidence-based guidance become an evidence-based directive in law or professional codes of conduct? Moreover, we wonder whether ignorance of evidence-based guidance would constitute a poor legal defence. In the UK, guidelines are introduced into courts by expert witnesses as evidence of accepted and customary standards of care, but cannot, as yet, be introduced as a substitute for expert testimony. However, in the USA a study has shown that guidelines play a relevant or pivotal part in the proof of negligence in 6–7 per cent of malpractice actions.[1] Presently, in medicine, evidence-based guidelines set normative standards such that departure from them may require explanation, but they do not constitute a *de facto* legal standard of care.[2]

The potential legal ramifications are crucial in evaluating the likely effects of evidence-based practice (EBP) on frontline social work practice. Returning to the scenario, had it not been for Graham McBeal's unexpected but forthright retort to the prosecuting solicitor, Suzy Taylor's professional credibility would have been brought into question. However, if Suzy had known about Graham's planned revenge on behalf of his sister, the evidence she would have required to reach a decision would have been based on entirely different parameters. That is, she would have needed research evidence on the likelihood of an older brother committing grievous bodily harm on a boy of a similar age, following an attack of a female sibling. It is highly unlikely that such an evidence base would have been available to Suzy, even if she had known of the planned attack in advance. More ludicrously, a randomized controlled trial (RCT) would certainly not have been available. Evidence-based guidance simply does not drill down this far, nor does it deal with chance or the complexity of scenarios such as this.

Issues of complexity and relevance have run consistently throughout this book. In various chapters we have defined evidence-based social work as entailing the mobilization of a specialist research infrastructure to guide a particular approach to practice which originated in evidence-based medicine. Evidence-based practice *becomes* evidence-based social work at the point that it *materializes, is performed and made durable in a more or less fixed set of locations within social work*, e.g., in social work agencies or professional cultures of social work practice. We have outlined the importance of diffusion theory and actor network theory in understanding the transportability of evidence-based practice *into* social work, based on a series of implementation or translation moves, to become 'evidence-based social work'. In doing so, we argued that producing evidence does not lead automatically to evidence-based social work. Hence that claims to be applying 'best available evidence' do not necessarily equate to evidence-based social work. Evidence-based social work is more complex, involving much more than what the social work practitioner does at the precise moment of decision-making. Most importantly, we have shown that evidence-based practice is an emergent phenomenon that has yet to be fully realized as 'evidence-based social work' and is unlikely to have an easy passage into social work settings, given the high degree of contestability about the relation between knowledge, evidence and information, what constitutes evidence-based practice, what counts as evidence and how it should be implemented. In Chapter 1, we showed that there are important distinctions between 'knowledge', 'evidence' and 'information' which suggested that these terms should be carefully considered and not used interchangeably or as a matter of convenience.

As we show below, our own position leans toward Davenport and Prusak's (1998: 10) widely accepted distinction between information, evidence and knowledge for social work, in providing the following 'pragmatic description' of knowledge in organizations:

> Knowledge is a fluid mix of framed experience, values, contextual information, and expert insight that provides a framework for evaluating and incorporating new experiences and information. It originates and is applied in the minds of knowers. In organizations, it often becomes embedded not only in documents or repositories but also in organizational routines, processes, practices, beliefs and norms.

This kind of pragmatic approach to knowledge can be translated in such a way that helps social workers to ask important questions. What does research to practice look and sound like in day-to-day working life? How is practical knowledge different from evidence and information? Where do I find it? How do I use it? What do we talk about when we talk about practice-based knowledge? In other words, what do I *do* on Monday morning when the phone starts ringing to help make the social work agency's use of knowledge more effective for service users (Ekbia and Hara 2008)?

Mobilizing knowledge in action

Research for practice

Our starting point in the conclusion to this book is to affirm that it is both reasonable and necessary for social workers to be able to understand and use research in their professional frontline practice: to know and understand 'what' evidence is out there. We regard the integration of research with practice as a central feature of professions such as social work. Knowing about the different kinds of social science, law and policy research that are available, and how to gain access to them and critically appraise them, is an increasingly necessary skill for social work practitioners to have. In this respect, we have advocated a form of pragmatic knowledge-based social work that incorporates critical inquiry and value perspectives. Enhancing the translation of research into practice is an important consideration for researchers, policy-makers, practitioners and service users alike. However, an important aim of this book has been to critically explore the extent to which the view that an evidence-based approach to social work implies that research is capable of generating knowledge that makes possible more effective interventions. We wished to examine whether this view on evidence-based practice could be sustained and to identify the conditions that would have to be met to make it possible, while exploring its strengths and limitations as a strategy for improving social work practice. More critically, we suggested that presently the case for the deployment of evidence-based practice in social work *does not satisfy or meet evidence-based practice's own internal criteria* for the admissibility of research. In plain terms, there is no 'gold standard' research evidence to prove conclusively that social work would effectively benefit from the implementation of evidence-based practice. There is no substantial evidence to vindicate its application and less still to justify implementation arguments from medical or health-related studies. With this in mind, we invited social work researchers and practitioners to consider whether evidence-based social work is an unnecessary distraction to the realities of frontline practice. We feel it is time for protagonists of evidence-based social work to concede that the internal criteria for admissible research are not being met in the recommendations being made for social work. We also think it is time that they accept that the gap between medical and social work research cannot be bridged in justifications for transfer models from one field to the other. Even if we had rigorous and valid evidence from a set of RCTs comparing representative samples of social work interventions in different fields and across different service user groups, this would still not meet the medical criteria for meta-analysis or research synthesis.

Social work is a risky business (Webb 2006) that is politically, economically and socially infused in a rapidly changing and complex environment in ways that are not susceptible to statistical generalizations or systematic review. There is inevitably a range of ideological stances involved in the agenda of those championing evidence-based practice that might impact badly on the frontline practitioners expected to implement it. The evidence offered by evidence-based protagonists is, in fact, interpretations that act as performatives (Latour 1996: 187). Its success is achieved by transforming the social work world in conformity with their perspective on this world. The proponents of evidence-based practice for social work need to acknowledge what has been accepted for a long time in the philosophy of sciences, that is, the role that the knowing investigator plays in constituting the world. They should not ignore the methodological irreducibility of their own perspective. If they do, the champions of evidence-based practice falsely stabilize their interpretations and end up creating a world for others that strongly resembles an absolute world with fixed and narrow reference points. Evidence-based practice thus comes to represent a 'closed system' rather than an open one. However, translations occur that strategically shift the evidence-based program from one side of the experimental continuum to some fuzzy middle ground. In Chapter 1, we explained how the evidence-based project necessarily gets more complicated because liberal advocates, such as Gambrill and Soydan, need to reinscribe *in it* whatever threatens to interrupt its course. This was referred to as a strategy of accommodation. The cascading effect of Gambrill's translations of appeasement, while trying to maintain consensus, abandons the rigour of positivist purists, such as Thyer, Sheldon and Lipsey, and thus ceases to authorize evidence-based practice in its experimental scientific guise.

As we argued in Chapter 5, in our examination of the UK House of Commons Selection Committee report, it is inevitable that professional judgement will always take priority over evidence in informing decision-making. Indeed, it seems to us that professional judgement is 'the gold standard' of evidence. Let us remind readers of what UK Chancellor of the Exchequer Alistair Darling reported to the Select Committee: '... there comes a time when you say, "You use your judgment." There could be other things where there is evidence that something works, and, for perfectly good policy reasons, we say it is not the thing we want to do' (Ev.72, Q1322), and the Selection Committee recommendation: 'It would be more honest and accurate to acknowledge the fact that while evidence plays a role in informing policy, decisions are ultimately based on a number of factors – including political expediency' (Appendix to House of Commons Select Committee Report 2007, Recommendation 35). Just as political expediency quite rightly plays a vital role in the decision-making processes of the Chancellor of the Exchequer, so it appropriately does in the day-to-day decisions of frontline social workers. Decision-making in social work will always entail a complex mix of life experience, professional judgement, heuristics, political expediency and research knowledge.

Evidence-based practice is not just about what the practitioner does

To return to the point we raised above regarding misconceptions within social work practice about 'what doing' evidence-based social work means, the standard definition of evidence-based practice derived from Sackett *et al.* (1996, 1997, 2000) does not lend itself readily to social work. No matter how clear the steps in the evidence-based practice approach are made, it is misleading to imply that evidence-based practice is merely something that behaviourally happens at the level of the practitioner, i.e., that it is merely about individual practitioners formulating practice questions and locating and using evidence to make practice decisions. Rubin's (2008: 7) more recent definition of evidence-based social work is a good example of a definition directly derived from Sackett *et al.*:

> EBP is a process for making practice decisions in which practitioners integrate the best research evidence available with their practice expertise and with client attributes, values, preferences, and circumstances. When those decisions involve selecting an intervention ... practitioners ... attempt to maximize the likelihood that their clients will receive the most effective intervention possible in light of ... the most rigorous scientific evidence available; practitioner expertise; client attributes, values, preferences, and circumstances; assessing for each case whether the chosen intervention is achieving the desired outcome; and if the intervention is not achieving the desired outcome, repeating the process of choosing and evaluating alternative interventions.

Interestingly, Rubin (2008) believes that evidence-based practice does not involve the mechanical application of interventions, as does the empirically supported treatment approach (Bledsoe *et al.* 2007), which is too narrow for social work practice. But for us, even Rubin's (2008) definition is limited. Hence we have proposed an alternative definition of evidence-based social work to show that what individual practitioners do takes place within a far broader networked context than that of the practitioner–service user interface:

> Evidence-based practice entails the mobilization of a broad – international – specialist research infrastructure that can – if translation procedures are put in place that directly address issues at the coalface – guide practitioners through particular interventions, support agencies in best practice governance and demonstrate positive outcomes for service users.

The evidence-based infrastructure has, thus far, focused on knowledge-building, in the process generating a burgeoning literature coming mainly from social work researchers, drawing on developments in, among other disciplines, psychology, education, criminal justice, social policy and social welfare more broadly. These researchers have focused on introducing evidence-based practice into social work education, especially in the USA, as we saw in Chapter 4. In the UK, there has been a great deal of activity at the policy level and with network-building, as we saw in Chapter 5. Despite these macro-level thrusts, evidence-based practice has failed to permeate the boundaries of social work practice, notwithstanding concerted efforts to develop a looser, more flexible and accommodating definition of evidence-based social work than is implied in Sackett *et al.*'s over-quoted source definition. Definitions of evidence-based social work advanced by various authors seem to be more mechanically focused around what Rubin (2008) calls the 'intervention perspective' and fail to sufficiently incorporate the strategic *process* of evidence-based networks and its interacting core elements of practice guidelines, practitioner expertise, client values and preferences, and available best evidence. Some erroneously see 'evidence-based social work' and 'evidence-based practice *in* social work' as being synonymous (Mullen, Shlonsky *et al.* 2005).

Gibbs (2003: 6), ahead of his time and writing at a juncture when evidence-based practice was almost alien to social work, emphasized an important point with great appeal to practitioners, which has somehow been lost in an over concern with empirically supported interventions, i.e., that it is a *process* which places the client first. He highlighted its impact, i.e., it forces 'evidence-based practitioners to adopt a process of lifelong learning that involves continually posing questions of *direct practical importance to clients*, searching objectively and efficiently for the current best evidence relative to each question, and taking appropriate action guided by evidence' (emphasis added). He emphasizes, too, that the notion of 'evidence' is not self-evident; it must be critically appraised (see discussion below).

What is common in most definitions is their attempt to persuade social workers to engage in 'research-based practice'. Notwithstanding our call for a much broader definition of pragmatic knowledge-based social work, what makes 'evidence-based practice in social work' or 'evidence-based social work' distinct is the comprehensiveness of the evidence-based practice approach and its attempt to move social workers beyond using research or evaluating their own practice in the style of the empirical-clinical practitioner approach, to being able to locate and critically appraise empirical evidence. Remember we maintain that evidence-based practice does not – and will not – eventuate without a comprehensive infrastructure supporting its translation into daily social work practice. By this we do not mean giving the practitioner a step-by-step approach but rather engaging with them on the complex cases of daily practice and the usefulness of and obstacles to evidence-based practice that they encounter. Claims that social workers are uninterested in or do not use research are most unhelpful in this endeavour. There needs to be empathic engagement about why this is so rather than blanket assumptions that there is something wrong with what social workers are doing. Empathy requires entertaining the idea that something might be wrong with the evidence-based practice approach which they are being called upon to apply.

Critical appraisal works both ways

A major problem is that much of the endorsement for evidence-based social work is being done without any concerted engagement with practitioners at the coalface and, ironically, without any evidence that evidence-based practice works. The major advocates promoting evidence-based practice in social work have an ethical obligation to practitioners to demonstrate empirically that what they are advocating works, i.e., 'how it works' in such a way that it will improve outcomes for service users. Actor network theory shows us that it is unlikely to translate to the practice coalface unless practitioners are convinced of its veracity and unless they are strongly supported in adopting and using an evidence-based practice approach. Practitioners can and should demand evidence that evidence-based practice works *for* social work.

Hence in this concluding chapter, we examine the implications of the evidence-based agenda from the social work practitioner's perspective. Our aim is to provide the practitioner with some critical skills for approaching calls for them to embrace evidence-based practice. We have already emphasized the importance of practitioners being cognizant of research-for-practice. It is important for social workers to keep up-to-date with the latest research, regardless of the approach they are taking. We must recognize that this is no small task for busy social workers with large caseloads, who are required to demonstrate in performance terms a quick turnaround, so that the case can be closed. We think it important for practitioners to grasp that, regardless of claims by major actors in promoting evidence-based practice, evidence cannot simply 'speak for itself' because the *meaning* of that evidence is of another order altogether. Much more is required than 'individual practitioners critically appraising available best evidence'. Those generating the evidence have an ethical obligation to ensure that it is 'best evidence', that the methodologies they use are sound and rigorous and suited to the problem under study. As Mark Lipsey (2003: 80) notes from his work on meta-analysis, 'Advice drawn from meta-analysis about what program characteristics most influence intervention outcomes and when methodological characteristics bias study findings about those outcomes, however, must be made very cautiously'.

Practitioners, too, need to be aware of debates about what constitutes evidence and whether 'best evidence' is that derived from RCTs – the 'gold standard' of evidence-based practice – or whether other forms of research also qualify, as we discussed in Chapter 2. Practitioners must be concerned, as well, about that way in which evidence is manipulated and contextualized under the aegis of regulation for greater efficiency, whether in the name of political expediency or of scientific truth. They have reason to criticize the artificial norms imposed upon frontline practice by regulators and the way in which diverse modes of professional decision-making are ignored by evidence-based practice, as we discussed in Chapter 6. In this spirit, practitioners must also critically appraise evidence-based social work itself. They should weigh up the arguments for and against evidence-based social work and not simply assume it as a given, as Sheldon suggests (see Chapter 5).

Cohen *et al.* (2004) have succinctly described the shortcomings of evidence-based practice, believing that: (i) it relies too heavily on empiricism and a narrow definition of evidence; (ii) ironically, it lacks any evidence of its own efficacy; (iii) it is of limited use for clients and service users; and (iv) it threatens the autonomy of the social worker or client relationship. Practitioners must, as we have attempted to do, politicize the ways of understanding the evidence network and the assumptions about evidence-based social work that have become common, particularly in certain quarters of the research and policy community.

Throughout this book we have pointed to the complexities of the evidence-based practice project, believing strongly that the case for or against evidence-based social work needs to be made both empirically and conceptually. There is nothing simple or linear about evidence-based practice. It is not just a matter of finding and applying evidence, or using evidence to make practice decisions. A critical stance is needed and practitioners need to understand that they are situated within an interlocking network which seeks to enrol them in the evidence-based project.

The practitioner's perspective

What then are the requirements and experiences of evidence-based social work from the practitioner's point of view? Research analysis and debate in social work about theoretical, conceptual and historical developments can, at times, seem remote from the realities and demands of practitioner experience and we do not wish to fall into that trap. Evidence-based discourse is a reality in policy, methodology and some practice interventions in social work. Social workers practising within the current context require a critical understanding of evidence-based social work in order to respond constructively. It has been our intention in this book to offer social workers not only a conceptual analysis of evidence-based practice, but also a resource that will be useful in practice. In Chapter 1, we challenged practitioners to view evidence-based practice not merely as a technique for or approach to practice but as being intrinsically tied to the cultural, policy and organizational environment in which practice happens. Throughout, we have tried to show that the way in which evidence is defined, how research is conducted and the connections between research and practice environments are influenced by historical developments and key actors in particular settings, with particular analyses in Chapters 4 and 5 on the USA, UK and the international scene.

So for social work practitioners moving into or embedded in settings where they are being entreated to use evidence-based practice, the first step is to investigate and establish how evidence is understood in that context, how research is practised, what is valued, who are the key players or actors, and how an evidence-based approach has taken shape in that context. They can use the information contained in the chapters of this book to critically appraise these parameters and, based on their critical analysis, may choose to work within the existing parameters or aim to establish themselves as key players in shaping where evidence-based social work in that particular context leads in the future. To this end, the opening chapter offers the practitioner some ways in which evidence-based practice has been conceptualized as a particular approach to practice, which rests on research that is conducted in a particular way (Chapter 2) and guidelines and protocols designed to guide practitioner decision-making. We urge practitioners to move the discussion beyond the simplistic view of the 'what works' agenda, with its focus on locating 'the best available evidence' for 'best practice', and note that grounds are needed for moral judgements such as these. They need, too, to raise questions about how knowledge for practice is being formalized by evidence-based practice actors within their particular professional context. Here they might be mindful of the way in which evidence-based practice has been translated into different international contexts, as outlined in Chapter 4, including the way in which it has developed in the UK, as discussed in Chapter 5. They also need to be aware of the limitations of the implementation model, discussed in Chapter 6, which places the onus of implementation on the individual practitioner when, as we argue, the knowledge translation model is a much more accurate framework for understanding implementation, which involves much more than the individual practitioner at the coalface. Remember, as we have noted in our definition, that evidence-based practice is the endpoint of a massive research, policy and practice infrastructure pushing the practitioner in a particular direction.

Implementation of evidence-based practice is not an automatic process of translation, given the myriad micro and macro factors that social workers need to work with in order to implement practices that are well supported by research evidence. These include cultural, strategic and environmental factors, as well as a range of personal and practical issues that can inhibit the implementation of an evidence-based practice approach. While practitioner skills – like interpersonal, teamwork, organizational, conflict resolution, negotiation, assessment, advocacy, lobbying and leadership skills – are helpful in working towards evidence-based practice at the personal, professional and organizational levels, a much broader understanding is needed. Understanding the broader context and issues involved in evidence-based practice enables critical appraisal. The more practitioners critique what is being asked of them, the better the outcome will be if evidence-based practice is, indeed, to work at the coalface. Social work practitioners need to document their experiences to build a bottom-up knowledge base – a mirror for the macro-level theorists and policy-makers to gaze into to see the extent to which the measures they are pushing are in fact achievable in practice.

Arenas of evidence-based practice

The frameworks for critical engagement with evidence-based practice offered in this book could be helpful for social workers in diverse practice arenas, including policy, multi-disciplinary and evidence-based teams and, most importantly, direct work with individuals and families, groups and communities.

The policy arena

'Evidence-based practice' has become a buzzword in many organizational and government policies relating to the provision of human services. Practitioners and researchers are required to identify and demonstrate evidence-based strategies as though this were an unambiguous and viable expectation. As we have shown, this is rarely, if ever, the case, given the complexities associated with identifying relevant, adequate and 'best' evidence for policy decision-making. Social workers who adopt an informed and critical perspective on evidence for human service practice will be able to engage in debates about how various types of knowledge, including evidence, may be useful in different contexts. They will understand and accept that informed and ethical judgements are, more often than not, made knowing that evidence is never absolute or complete but must suffice given that it is the best available for now. They will understand, too, that there are dangers in assuming that evidence from reputable sources can be translated uncritically, uniformly and automatically into different policy contexts, especially since an evidence-based practice approach is contingent not only on evidence but also on practitioner judgement and client values. Rather than bowing to a superior scientific authority, the social worker with an informed and critical perspective on evidence-based practice will be confident to examine and challenge the assumptions about evidence and simplistic notions of 'best practice', while being able to inform clients on what is known about their particular problem at that point in time. On making judgements about adequate and appropriate evidence, the social worker is then in a position to work simultaneously at a macro level to develop policies and programs, knowledgeable about the micro and macro factors that enable policies to become practices with the potential to effect a real and positive influence on clients and communities.

But they need, too, to understand what drives policy agendas. Evidence-based policy implies that it is research, that policies must be based on the best research evidence available at the time. However, politically savvy social workers know the idealism of this claim and they know that public policy-makers ignore their voting public at their peril (Sherman 2003). They are unlikely to make or implement new policies, no matter what the latest research says, if it is going to cause a public outcry. Here social workers are always caught because the interests of their clients are often unpopular with the voting public, who are always loathe to support increased resources for their marginalized clients whom, more often than not, they see as dependent through their own doing. The voting public is not always sympathetic to social work causes and shows little regard for critical social work's structural understanding of social problems.

Besides the voting public, however, are the social researchers who generate the evidence for policy-makers. Sherman (2003) points to some evidence of mistrust here and Hammersley (2003) alerts us to the competing interests of social researchers and public policy-makers. These factors constitute a major obstacle for evidence-based practice. Let us begin with Sherman (2003: 7–8), who notes that:

> ... a double challenge in government ... to *produce* more evidence and to make better *use* of what evidence there is [and] ... social science is failing government on both challenges ... due to weak research designs, and too little social science evidence is presented in a way that allows government to assess the risk of bias (emphasis in the original).

For Hammersley (2003), this situation arises because the purpose of social research is to produce new knowledge about social problems rather than *usable information per se*. Policy-makers are more likely to trust social researchers that supply them with evidence that suits their purposes. They are likely to see researchers who produce unpalatable findings as obstructive and unhelpful. There is always the likelihood that the findings of research might not be favourable for policy-makers or even practitioners, and that they might be unpopular, as was Joel Fischer's groundbreaking work on the effectiveness of social casework in the 1970s, discussed in Chapter 4.

As Sherman (2003) noted, governments are reluctant to rely on social science evidence which they consider to be biased, especially where ideological differences pertain. Such concerns cloud the production and integrity of *evidence*. However, whether evidence 'leads or misleads policy decisions may depend on intelligent consumers understanding the *logical* distinctions rather than *ideological* divisions in the methods and epistemologies of contemporary social science' (Sherman 2003: 7, emphasis in the original). Sherman (2003) sees the importance of policy-makers as consumers having a clear understanding of research methodology. He says that because social researchers and academics are often seen as being ideologically motivated, US policy-makers are increasingly turning to private research enterprises and consultants, internet searches, and expert think-tanks, for evidence. This creates further confusion, because often what is presented as research, especially from the internet and think-tanks, is often *information-based* rather than *research-based*. Strictly, then, it is not evidence derived from reliable data based on rigorous, objective, replicable, valid, scientific research studies, as discussed in Chapter 2. As we have seen, the findings of systematic and rigorous research are often complex and difficult to translate directly into usable knowledge and there is the ever-present danger that unpopular findings will be ignored. In other words, social researchers, like Hammersley (2003), believe that the type of research which policy-makers seek is often aimed at justifying or legitimating rather than questioning or critiquing their policy agendas. For Hammersley, researchers are not merely suppliers of information to suit powerful stakeholders – such as politicians, the voting public and the media – in the stakeholders' quest for evidence-based policy. However, neither are policy-makers mere users of information or research. There is a circular argument at work here, because the extent to which policy-makers use evidence depends largely on whether or not they trust social scientists and their research methods (Sherman 2003). Social scientists' inability to agree on which scientific methods are most appropriate for informing policy thwarts their propensity to contribute to the evidence-based policy project.

To avoid the dangers of information-based policy-making and to overcome disagreements among social researchers, the US Federal Government made a groundbreaking decision that only research based on RCTs of its educational reform program, ushered in by the 'No Child Left Behind' Act, would be funded. Thus it went to the opposite extreme in stipulating the particular research methods to be used in pursuing answers to major policy questions in education, as the government defines them. Not surprisingly, it has come under severe criticism from social researchers, most notably proponents of qualitative inquiry, such as Cannella and Lincoln (Cannella and Lincoln 2004; Lincoln and Cannella 2004). They believe that this move effectively excludes alternative epistemologies or rival social understandings and permits the Federal Government to usurp the roles of professional disciplines and communities, limiting the voices that are heard in policy circles, and narrowing broad peer review to a small band of federally 'approved' reviewers. They warn that, far from assuring objective knowledge about social programs, such constriction assures a tight oligarchy of researchers and new knowledge gatekeepers, with few insights from alternative forms of scholarly inquiry.[3] They anticipate the consequences of the complete application of evidence-based policy as a process of formalization which effectively locks out other players and diverse methodologies. In such a regulatory mode, government policy closes down research avenues within academic institutions and research organizations which attempt any form of critical or broader social and political analysis. This is of even more concern for some who believe that policy has been a key driver of evidence-based practice from the outset and who believe that the evidence-based policy model raises questions of survival for professions and social service organizations within managerialist, economic rationalist environments (Morago 2006; Trinder 2000). Seeing how the major Western nations influence one another *vis-à-vis* policy development, one might well wonder how far away similar initiatives were in the UK, Australia and beyond. The formation of the Campbell Collaboration – or C2 – in the USA, with its strong contingent of educationists, was influential in this federal decision. Robert Boruch, the first chair of C2, served as a member of the committee that produced the National Research Council (2002) report edited by Shavelson and Towne, which emphasized RCTs. Other strong proponents of RCTs on the committee included Eric Hanushek, an economist at the Hoover Institute at Stanford.

In the UK, as we saw in Chapter 5, evidence-based practice is policy driven in a different way. Evidence-based policy is not necessarily about research informing policy so much as the evidence-based practice agenda being driven by policy-makers, research leaders and government civil servants with political agendas. Hence the macro-service infrastructure created by government has been a key driver in evidence-based practice in the UK.

It is helpful for practitioners to understand these broader political dynamics at work in shaping evidence-based policy and practice, as well as research agendas, as Sherman (2003), writing in the USA, and Hammersley (2003), writing in the UK, show. These background factors inevitably influence what happens in the organizational contexts in which practitioners work.

The social service organization

The service sector is complex and beset by issues of financial viability, interorgan-izational relations, administrative systems, including computer technology, as well as micro-level client–worker issues. As we have outlined above, the cultural climate in which the practitioner works is a major factor in the translation of evidence to practice (see Figure 7.1). We know from organizational and management research that a climate of trust, openness, sharing, collegiality, support for innovation, valuing of critical perspectives, coaching and mentoring, is an invaluable part of the focus on *process* which Rubin (2008) says is lacking in relation to evidence-based social work. Research also demonstrates that 'the development of databases that capture knowledge increases availability of knowledge to employees' (Ekbia and Hara 2008: 17). Both awareness and availability of knowledge are important, and possibly agencies should employ experienced librarians whose job it is to constantly search for, locate and disseminate evidence in the agency's field of practice. Hence the social service organization must provide the physical and supportive resources for practitioners to access evidence, i.e., the time to do so, the technology needed, the training to support the use of the technology, coaching in using it, and so on.

The multi-disciplinary practice arena

Multi-disciplinary practice offers a rich and holistic response to the needs of service users, but can also be a source of conflict as different perspectives and bodies of knowledge clash. One such source of conflict is around what is valued as research and as evidence for practice. Different professional disciplines are concerned with different practice questions, which may lend themselves to particular notions of evidence or research designs. Social workers operating in multi-disciplinary contexts will benefit from an understanding of the strengths and limitations of different research designs in gathering evidence for particular practice questions. In such contexts they will also gain an appreciation that all professional disciplines have formalized and adopted particular bodies of knowledge as a result of contextual influences, historical developments, professional values and key actors in the process. We have provided a description of what the process has been in social work and recognized that this may be somewhat different for other professions. Medical professions and the type of treatments doctors use might certainly be more amenable to scientific research, especially where drug trials are concerned, than are 'social' professions like teaching, law and social work, which often rely on contested evidence, evidence from a variety of perspectives and so on. For example, in our child protection scenario at the outset, Suzy Taylor, the social worker, had to make a professional judgement despite many different interpretations of what was happening in the McBeal family from teachers, neighbours, parents, siblings, the prosecuting solicitor, and so on. This is not to deny the skill of medical practice and the human side, which evidence-based medicine encompasses in the notions of 'professional expertise' and 'client preference'. It is rather to realistically appraise the accessibility of the phenomena with which social workers deal to strict RCT study.

Evidence-based teams

Social work is inherently a team performance. We have found very little research or modelling on the various merits or disadvantages of adopting an evidence-based team approach to applying research to practice. This is rather surprising, given that current social work literature often cites communication breakdown and teamwork failures as primary threats to delivering effective interventions for service users.[4] As we observe below in our discussion of the types of evidence that practitioners use (see Figure 7.1), the culture of the evidence-based team cannot be overlooked. Notwithstanding that different disciplines and professions might have different views on evidence, organizational environments which create an atmosphere of collegial sharing are most likely to produce efficient, evidence-based teams.

- Financial and annual reports
- Agency documents (policy and mission statements, letters, memos, emails, and so on)
- Interviews and discussions with managers, colleagues and service users
- Recognition received for prior successes from supervisors, colleagues and service users
- Cultural issues, such as the way knowledge is shared within the organization, levels of managerial and collegial trust, the supportiveness of the work environment, and so on
- Standardized methods across different offices, locations and projects
- Cooperation in learning and sharing experiences for building a shared 'we are all in this together' identity
- Usability or widespread use of information and whether it is part of accepted agency practice
- Efficiency – saving money and time while still offering quality services and producing tangible benefits for service users
- Participant enthusiasm – practitioners are more likely to use evidence which others are using and which is commonly the focus of their case discussions
- Productivity – practitioners are likely to value evidence which increases productive outcomes for service users
- Relationships between and with managers, colleagues and service users – individuals in the practitioner's social network – are likely to have a major influence on what becomes culturally accepted as evidence
- Knowledge-sharing is crucial to the cultural embedding of evidence
- Availability of knowledge and access to knowledge are equally important to the cultural embedding of evidence, which, in turn, determines the ease or not of knowledge transfer
- Intervention, particularly support for practitioners attempting to implement empirically supported interventions. Practitioners are more likely to use interventions with proven effectiveness, which may or may not be empirically supported. Thus the degree of support and guidance received will determine practitioner willingness to try new innovations. A focus on process is essential.
- Anecdotal comments or the power of word-of-mouth cannot be overlooked in daily practice
- Measuring intellectual capital or knowledge assets is important if a culture of continuous improvement in practitioner knowledge and competency is to be achieved
- Increasing revenues – nothing cements a practice better than the continued funding which comes from the work being done
- Trust and a climate of openness are essential for the testing of new innovations. Critical discussions of EBP and the smoothing of its path for translation to practice can only happen in an environment of trust, openness and sharing
- Support and recognition from CEOs, management and colleagues, and service user satisfaction, are powerful sources of evidence for practitioners in their daily practice
- Recognition for knowledge-creation efforts and sharing of information garnered, via discussion and debate, are likely to smooth the path of EBP

Figure 7.1 Pragmatic sources for social workers.

Adapted from Ekbia and Hara (2008: 25–26).

Direct work with clients, groups and communities

As we showed in relation to social work practice in Germany and Scandinavia in Chapter 4, social workers are eager to retain the critically reflective nature of their practice and believe that their critical reflection skills equip them with many and varied abilities – to appraise research and examine the applicability of findings to different contexts, to reflect upon personal and contextual factors and to make well-considered, ethical practice decisions – all of which are features of evidence-based social work. According to this understanding, evidence-based social work may be seen as a considered and reflective approach to practice that may be used to guide social work education and professional development. But as we have shown throughout this book, it is much more complex than this. It is about a particular type of knowledge-generation, in particular contexts which may or may not sustain professional and organizational groupings in social work. There is a great deal of sensitivity to the loss of professional autonomy as part of the evidence-based practice agenda, as seen in Chapter 5. Evidence-based practice, as we have argued, is not just about establishing individual approaches to practice and identifying how social work can best serve the needs of clients, groups and communities. We have argued that Sackett *et al.*'s (1997, 2000) definition of evidence-based practice as the 'conscientious, explicit and judicious use of current best evidence in making decisions' does not serve social work well. Crucially it assumes that individual practitioners make clinical decisions about individual patients and totally overlooks the broad research infrastructure and macro-policy environment driving a particular approach to clinical decision-making to the exclusion of others.

The practice scenarios which follow demonstrate that practitioner decision-making is only one element of the evidence-based practice approach, which takes place in a process that involves the assessment of complex individual, family and community problems within equally complex organizational, policy and social environments. Social work interventions are not directed only toward individuals, but also toward the systems and networks impacting upon individual lives. While the future of evidence-based social work relies upon building a bank of knowledge derived from sound research evidence of effectiveness for individual practice, it also entails mobilizing systems of governance. The frontline practitioner cannot make sound decisions about effective practice unless supported by an infrastructure which:

1 produces a range of international, national and local information drawn from systematic research that can be integrated in making well-considered judgements for practice. Experimental findings, descriptions of the impacts of a range of interventions in particular cultural and organizational environments and well-documented client experience all constitute relevant information for practice.
2 synthesizes diverse research findings and develops best practice guidelines suited to particular cultural and organizational contexts. This necessarily entails coordination between professional and governance systems, with input from consumer or service user groups.

3   generates policies and resources to support practitioners and managers in the implementation of the evidence-based practice approach and best practice guidelines. Best practice guidelines serve little purpose for practitioners involved in bottom-up, evidence-based decision-making when top-down managerial policies and systems are not in touch with everyday practice realities.

4   supports educational and professional development programs which take cognisance of the ethical principles that guide social work practice and research and instil a critically reflective approach to practice incorporating not just hyper-reflexivity and self-reflection but also well-developed skills in the appraisal, synthesis and application of research findings.

Evidence-based practice offers a framework for social workers to study and improve their practice and to develop empirical evidence on the value of social work intervention. Evidence-based practice highlights that continual improvement of the quality of services is an obligation we owe to the clients and communities we serve. Evidence-based social work has been shaped by the prevailing values and ethics of the profession and the theories on which it draws, which we have grouped, following Plath (in Gray and Webb 2008), into a four-pronged analytic framework comprising positivist, pragmatic, political and postmodern influences. We have argued that evidence-based social work is an amalgam of scientific – positivist and interpretivist – practical and political considerations. We have proposed that there is a range of ways in which social workers access, appraise or interpret, engage with and apply evidence for practice, determined largely by the particular social, political and organizational context in which they practice. Some of these contexts, such as the health system, have better-developed infrastructures for evidence-based practice than do others, such as small, community-based organizations, as the following case scenarios show.

Evidence-based social work in action

The following scenarios show how evidence-based social work approaches can be construed in a practice context. Rather than offering a step-by-step process to follow, the scenarios illustrate how evidence-based social work is dependent on local, situated knowledge and needs to be negotiated in particular contexts, highlighting the benefits it may accrue and also the significant challenges it presents.

Susan is a social worker in an adolescent mental health service that provides services to young people with eating disorders and their families. There is a strong medical and research culture within the service provided by the public health system. Evidence shows that eating disorders, such as anorexia nervosa and bulimia, often result in severe illness, long-term physiological ailments and, at times, death. The client group comprises young people who, free of the illness, are generally high achieving and productive. There is a strong imperative to identify treatment interventions that work in dealing with eating disorders. Susan is part of a multi-disciplinary team, which has adopted a particular treatment approach – called the Maudsley approach – that is well supported by large clinical trials and has a strong international research base, with new studies building further evidence of the effectiveness of this intervention. Hence the treatment approach has gained prominence at international conferences and in research publications. On the basis of this evidence, Susan feels confident about the potential for her work, as part of the multi-disciplinary team, to have positive outcomes for clients of the service. However, she is concerned that there are always a few clients who withdraw from the service. Sometimes the families let the service know that they cannot commit to what is required of them in the treatment regime. Susan decides to examine the evidence more closely and finds that all of the randomized controlled trials (RCTs) on the outcomes of this treatment reported a significant subject attrition rate. Motivated by a concern for the needs of treatment dropouts whom she defines as a minority and marginalized group, she searches a range of international online databases and gathers information on alternative treatment approaches in an effort to find ways to engage with and help young people and families who drop out of the service. The research findings she locates are less authoritative and definitive about the outcomes than the RCTs supporting this dominant treatment mode. Nonetheless, these studies offer useful qualitative and explanatory information about the factors that contribute to young people discontinuing treatment. Susan has also gathered material on other treatment models that seem to have achieved some positive outcomes and suggest that they may be more appealing to those people who withdraw from treatment. She advocates within the service for the needs of clients who do not suit the dominant treatment mode. It takes persistence and skills in negotiating, lobbying and arguing a well-evidenced case, but eventually the adolescent mental health service agrees to the implementation of innovative strategies to improve client engagement and the introduction of an alternative treatment option to the clients who withdraw from the mainstream intervention.

This scenario shows the limitation in the empirically supported treatment approach and why we need evidence-based practice, which is the approach Susan uses. She shifts the focus from the effectiveness of intervention for those individuals who complete treatment to the effectiveness of the service overall to the presenting client group. She then institutes a search, motivated by her social work values of inclusiveness, to identify an intervention which might re-engage young people who have dropped out of treatment. This case scenario demonstrates quite clearly that evidence-based social work is not exclusively about treatment effectiveness. The social worker used her clinical judgement and critical appraisal skills to effect change in the organizational setting where she works. But this is only the beginning, for she now has to build evidence that the alternative intervention which she has located from the research data indeed proves more effective for the client group she has identified. Alongside the evidence about 'what is the best treatment for anorexia nervosa or bulimia', she also posed the question 'Why are clients dropping out of treatment and how might they be re-engaged in the service?' She thus extended evidence-based social work beyond the way of the empirically supported treatment approach.

The Northside Family Support Service is a non-government organization that relies on government funding to provide home visiting, referral and case-management services to families with complex needs. Staff members in the service have made determined efforts to locate evidence about the types of interventions that are most effective in achieving positive outcomes for parents and children. Drawing on international practice research databases, best practice guidelines and internal evaluations, the service has developed its own best practice principles for responding to families with particular presenting issues. The reality of daily practice in the organization, however, is that families often present in a crisis and, while a particular type of service response is indicated, there are insufficient resources to support this evidence-based intervention. Attempts to refer families to specialist services are met with long waiting times, closed books or rigid eligibility criteria (e.g., absence of substance use). While intensive home support may be indicated, resource constraints within the service result in only minimal support being offered. Despite having developed a well-informed evidence base for practice, the Northside Service is finding that improvements for families have been difficult to demonstrate to the government funding body. They are faced with presenting an evidence-based case to justify their ongoing funding. They believe that the problem does not lie with the quality of their service but with the lack of resources, an uncoordinated service network and the punitive policy environment in which they operate. Without any concrete evidence on the effectiveness of their service, the family support workers at Northside cannot argue convincingly for continued funding. They are certain that any systematic empirical investigation will demonstrate convincingly the inadequacy of the funding policy, but they are not in a position to undertake such a study.

It is clear from this scenario that evidence of effectiveness is essential in making the economic claim for the survival of this service. Evidence can be used as an economic device to justify financial decision-making. The agency workers have interpreted evidence-based practice to mean locating available research, literature and guidelines for best practice in services similar to their own. Many services, like Northside, are faced with a lack of evidence that is specific to their context and a lack of resources to conduct their own research. The guidelines they have identified have not proved useful to them because they have not had adequate resources to implement the evidence-based guidance they indicate. The question 'How might we best use our resources to achieve the best possible outcomes for our clients?' was not one that they could answer with the available evidence. Efficient data management systems within the organization would enable them to determine the most pressing needs of their clients, the type of crises that precipitate requests for service, and so on. Such concrete data constitute a powerful base on which to build a proposal for further funding. But if it were possible for this small organization to implement such systems, it would result in even fewer resources being available to assist clients. To bolster this demand-side data, the agency could institute a program evaluation to follow up clients after they have received services, to assess whether or not their service was effective. By this time, the family support service would have become a research organization. There would be no need to eliminate ineffective practices, as there would be none to eliminate. All agencies operate within financial constraints. The demand for services will always exceed the supply. Evidence-based social work is a process, not a single event like locating best practice guidelines or an intervention that works. It involves locating research data on the most effective ways in which to render social support, even if this means locating evidence that social support is always ameliorative and never curative. But it is unreasonable to expect poorly funded organizations to provide services, evaluate and generate evidence on the effectiveness of those services, and then use this evidence to justify their continued existence. The motivation in such circumstances can be to keep one's position safe, rather than to seek out alternative interventions that are more effective. It would be more appropriate for research on service effectiveness to be conducted comprehensively by a coordinating authority, if this were to offer real guidance for practice. Otherwise evidence becomes little more than a tool in a political battle for resources, which can divert attention away from the adequacy of government funding to implement practice interventions that are well supported by the evidence.

José works for the Ministry for Family and Community Services in a country that is beginning to develop a government service response to child protection. He obtained a UK social work qualification and during his studies was exposed to the UK child protection system, which is far more developed than that in his own country. He sees his role as being to facilitate the development of systems and services that will result in a reduction of physical abuse and neglect of children. Building on knowledge gained from his studies, he identifies the types of interventions that have the strongest evidence for effective outcomes. His efforts to build this evidence base have been frustrating. While international practice evidence networks are accessible on the internet, internet access is slow and unreliable. The process of locating evidence is very time consuming. Many of the studies and systematic reviews he locates are not relevant, as they involve therapeutic interventions that require trained therapists, who are not available in his country. Other studies and best practice guidelines that he identifies are so entrenched in particular organizational and procedural contexts that they offer little that can be transferred to this setting. José does, however, identify a few programs that are well supported by research evidence and seem achievable. His efforts to implement these programs in local communities are, however, met with strong resistance both from community members and local administrators. After repeated, frustrated attempts, he decides to start where the local community is and reverts to a community development approach. He spends time getting to know people in the community and talks with them about their ideas on parenting, child maltreatment and strategies to improve their situation. While he draws on some of the knowledge and ideas he has gained from his review of the research, the process he engages in results in community education and support networks that are indigenous and appropriate to the local cultural context.

Given the positivistic underpinnings of certain evidence-based approaches to social work, we can discern how they rest heavily on the technologies of modern Western society, or what Gadamer called 'techne' and Habermas 'technical rationality' (see Chapter 1). Questions remain about their cross-national applications and cultural relevance. Rather than posing the question of 'How might I transport child protection models from the UK?', the question José needed to pose was 'What is the most culturally appropriate approach to practice here?'. Then he would have tried to locate evidence of effective community engagement strategies rather than evidence of Western child protection practice. The evidence-based practice approach highlights the importance of client preferences and values in combination with practitioner knowledge, expertise and judgement. José realized that strong evidence for effective child protection practice in the UK was not transferable to his own country. Instead, José's next search for evidence will stem directly from what he learns from local communities and involve community development principles and skills in interpersonal engagement and empathy.

These case studies demonstrate the potential significance of evidence but they also illustrate the complexity of variables involved in different events and decisions and that much more than evidence guides frontline social work practice. More accurately, evidence sits within a wider body of practice knowledge, which social workers use pragmatically in making professional judgements. It would seem to us, then, that social work rests on a pragmatism within which evidence is situated and combined with a range of other complex factors.

Pragmatic approach to social work

We discussed in Chapter 3 and noted above that pragmatic knowledge is practitioner centred and interested in defining the appropriate 'situated knowledge', i.e., it is grounded in practical, pragmatic purposes and how we use communication to reach common or shared solutions to practical problems. Similarly, it is grounded in locating meaningful evidence – evidence that we can use. Habermas's pragmatism is helpful here since it rests on communicative action and aims to provide tools for reaching decisions through rational discussion, i.e., through communication to reach shared understanding. An important part of his communicative action involves this common search for meaning.

Habermas's communicative approach also enables practitioners to pay attention to the power issues involved in evidence-based processes and strategies. Rather than top-down, policy-driven approaches to promulgating evidence-based practice, a pragmatic communicative approach seeks to engage the end users in the process of reaching shared decisions and understandings of the meaning of evidence and in devising appropriate care pathways for its translation into practice. Inevitably, it would take account of the real-life, day-to-day issues and problems which practitioners face and it would involve reversing the blackboxing which has occurred in policy-driven or other top-down regulatory approaches to evidence-based social work that have resulted in 'one size fits all' models. As Ekbia and Hara (2008: 21) note, 'blackboxing tends to cover the paths that have led to the final outcome, the choices that were made along the way, the options that were abandoned, the costs that were incurred, and so on'. By opening the black box, as it were – by asking how the guidelines were made, what kind of studies the research source involved, the nature of the findings, the methods used, the values of the researchers, and so on – practitioners not only bring a critical perspective to bear on the evidence but also add their voice to the discussion. A critical perspective seeks 'a balanced and clear account of the inner mechanisms, hidden costs, untried paths, and available options' (Ekbia and Hara 2008: 22) to the evidence-based practitioner. In the spirit of this 'critical perspective', reversing the blackboxing requires knowing who the human actors are in the evidence-based network: the policy-makers, executives, managers, information officers and trade publishers, as well as the academic researchers, information technology professionals, employees and scholarly journals that are promoting it. Also required is an awareness of these actors' different motivations, interests, understandings and commitments in furthering the evidence-based practice project. From an actor network perspective, practitioners might ask:

1 Which actors are involved?
2 Whose version of evidence is being considered?
3 Which actors need to be convinced in order for the evidence-based project to succeed?
4 Which ones should be isolated, neutralized, or dragged along?
5 What are the mobilization strategies of different actors?
6 What stage in the process are they up to?

Furthermore, practitioners should also be aware that often the 'success stories' claimed by the promoters are themselves instances of blackboxing. This is especially the case in the professional literature on the alleged benefits or success of evidence-based practice, rarely supported by empirical evidence. From this critical, pragmatic perspective, practitioners can bring their direct experience to bear on what might have become an abstract process of theorizing and researching far removed from the practice coalface. Let us reflect briefly on what knowledge-based practitioners might use on a daily basis. Here we include managers and frontline social workers.

In mobilizing knowledge for action, it is essential that we engage with the conventional sources of knowledge for practitioners in their daily practice, so as to see how strictly defined evidence might be translated into the culture of the practice environment. Davenport (in Ekbia and Hara 2008: 20) refers to these conventional knowledge sources as 'mundane knowledge', i.e., 'those aspects that relate to the local interactions of individuals within a physical and social environment' (*ibid.*: 11), which managers must take seriously.

Clearly, a pragmatic approach must take into account these locally contingent considerations if practitioners are to be convinced by the evidence-based practice project. But even more importantly, they must focus on the *process* of translation, i.e., the way in which it is done – the 'how' of translating evidence to practice rather than the 'what' of that knowledge being most strongly promoted at any given time. Social workers and case managers might consider:

1 how the knowledge to get work done is *presented and appropriated* in our organization;
2 how *structured interaction* might contribute to the management and dissemination of knowledge of daily practice;
3 whether persistent practices for mundane knowledge management emerge through *problem-based or scenario-based learning* strategies.

These are practical questions which start with 'how things are done around here', all of which are crucial considerations in the obligatory passage of evidence into practice. As the classic social work maxim says, 'we start where the practitioner is'.

'This ain't reality TV'

'This ain't reality TV!' yells Jack Nicholson – who plays mobster Costello in the movie *The Departed* – to the Irish hoodlum underling who has bungled the dumping of a dead body. Faced with some of the grimmest socio-economic circumstances, social workers are probably in one of the best positions to understand that reality doesn't resemble fiction. Frontline practice in the recovery houses of Philadelphia, the high-rise flats of south London, the tenement schemes of Dundee, or the shack-dweller towns of Durban is much closer to Costello's mobster world than it is to a scientific research laboratory or university research centre (Fairbanks 2008). Indeed, there is something about certain claims made for evidence-based practice that resemble fiction and even feel like a 'reality TV' show. The label 'reality TV' begs the question, 'How real is what we see?' The answer, of course, is, 'Not at all.' As Colin Sparks (2007) notes, 'what we see is a highly-constructed artefact rather than a slice of "real life"'. As with the experimentalist, observational techniques count for everything. In the infamous *Big Brother* reality TV show, the people we get to 'observe' are the product of an elaborate process of selection. Everything hangs together on the casting, to which scripting and editing come a close second. The evidence is commodified and any reference back to the source of the real-life event is lost. Toni Johnson-Woods (2002) notes that, to achieve dramatic narratives, the producers ruthlessly edit the raw footage: 'For example, in the first Australian series 182,750 hours of material were edited down to 70 hours of television' (cited in Sparks 2007: unpaginated). Does this not feel a little like the procedures involved in systematic reviews and good practice guidelines or protocols, whereby evidence-based practice is an edited selection of shots that are scripted for the practitioner? Just like reality TV, evidence-based practice uses real events, people and situations but chooses which bits to convey and manipulates them to produce an outcome. The process is contrived. The installation of guidelines and protocols capturing every moment of frontline decision, as with the cameras in the *Big Brother* house, has obvious parallels with the spread of closed-circuit television (CCTV) through the public spaces of the contemporary world. Social workers are recruited as scripted, edited participants in the evidence-based game. Professional creativity and autonomy are subordinated to the commands of the evidence-based director. The richness of frontline practice becomes reified in this artificially constructed world of quasi-science. The conformity demanded by evidence-based protocols means that, like the participants in *Big Brother*, social workers must abandon their professional autonomy and leave their own judgement at the door of the tightly surveilled house. Audience ratings are equivalent to the 'gold standard' RCTs, in that these are all that really count. As with *Big Brother*, the levels of scripted intervention increase as the show progresses. Evidence-based practice, while applying a sliding scale of 'factuality' to decisions, imagines a move for social work away from messy realities and more tightly framed around performance. This is a far cry from the harsh realities of street-level poverty, survival tactics, drugs and narcotics, family violence and abuse, and so on, that are ever-present in the difficult and often stressful judgements of social workers in how best to intervene. Evidence-based practice offers no challenge at all to these conditions and, indeed, its structure and method may well be replicating some of the most pernicious effects of 'technological reasoning' in advanced capitalist societies.

Notes

1 Hyams *et al.* (1995). Practice guidelines and malpractice litigation: a two way street. *Annals of Internal Medicine*, 22, 450–455.
2 Hurwitz, B. (2004). How does evidence based guidance influence determinations of medical negligence? *British Medical Journal*, 329, 1024–1028.
3 http://www.aaup.org/AAUP/pubsres/academe/2004/ND/BR/ndlinc.htm
4 http://www.rip.org.uk/changeprojects/documents/realteams/1evidencebased.pdf

References

Abbott, A. (1988). *The system of professions: an essay on the division of expert labor.* Chicago: University of Chicago Press.

Agrawal, A. (1995). Dismantling the divide between indigenous and scientific knowledge. *Development and Change*, 26, 413–439.

Agrawal, A. (2005). *Environmentality, technologies of government and the making of subjects.* Durham: Duke University Press.

Ainsworth, F. and Hansen, P. (2005). Evidence-based social work practice: A reachable goal? In Bilson, A. (ed.). *Evidence-based practice in social work.* London: Whiting & Birch.

Akiyama, K. and Buchanan, A. (2007). A comparison between Japanese and British research papers in key academic journals. *International Social Work*, 50(2), 255–264.

Akrich, M., Callon, M. and Latour, B. (2002a). The key to success in innovation Part II: the art of interessement. *International Journal of Innovation Management*, 6(2), 187–206.

Akrich, M., Callon, M. and Latour, B. (2002b). The key to success in innovation Part II: the art of choosing good spokespersons. *International Journal of Innovation Management*, 6(2), 207–225.

Allan, J., Pease, B. and Briskman, L. (2003). *Critical social work.* Crows Nest: Allen and Unwin.

Asscher, J.J., Dekovié, M., van Laan, P.H., Prins, P.J.M. and van Arum, S. (2007). Implementing randomized experiments in criminal justice settings: an evaluation of multi-systemic therapy in the Netherlands. *Journal of Experimental Criminology*, 3(2) 113–129.

Atherton, C.R. and Bolland, K.A. (2003). Postmodernism: a dangerous illusion, *International Social Work*, 45(4), 421–433.

Auslander, G.K. (2000). Social work research and evaluation in Israel. *Journal of Social Work Research and Evaluation*, 1, 17–34.

Austin, D. (1999). A report on progress in the development of research resources in social work. *Research on Social Work Practice*, 9, 673–707.

Austin, D. (1992). Findings of the NIMH [National Institute of Mental Health] task force on social work research. *Research on Social Work Practice*, 2(3), 312.

Austin, D.M. (1991). *Building social work knowledge for effective services and policies: a plan for research development.* Washington, DC: Task Force on Social Work Research, National Institute of Mental Health.

Bailey, R. and Brake, M. (1975). *Radical social work.* London: Edward Arnold.

Balas, E.A. and Boren, S.A. (2000). Managing clinical knowledge for health care improvement. *Yearbook of Medical Informatics.* Bethesda, MD: National Institute of Mental Health.

Barber, J. (2008). What evidence-based practice is. In White, B.W. (volume editor). *Comprehensive handbook of social work and social welfare: the profession of social work, Volume 1*. New Jersey: John Wiley and Sons, Inc.

Barlow, D.H. and Hersen, M. (1984). *Single case experimental designs: strategies for studying behavior change*. New York: Pergamon Press.

Barratt, M. (2003). Organizational support for evidence-based practice within child and family social work: a collaborative study. *Child and Family Social Work*, 8, 143–150.

Bellamy, J., Bledsoe, S.E. and Traube, D. (2006). The current state of evidence-based practice in social work: a review of the literature and qualitative analysis of expert interviews. *Journal of Evidence-Based Social Work*, 3(1), 23–48.

Bergin, A.E. and Garfield S.L. (eds). (1971). *Handbook of psychotherapy and behavior change: an empirical analysis*. New York: Wiley.

Bergman, M.M. (2008). *Advances in mixed methods research: theories and applications*. London: Sage.

Bergmark, A. and Lundström, T. (2008). Evidensfrågan och socialtjänsten: om socialarbetares inställning till en vetenskapligt grundad praktik (The evidence issue and the social services: on social workers' attitudes (point of view) to a practice based on science). *Socionomens Forskningssupplement*, 21, 5–14.

Bergmark, A. and Lundström, T. (2007). Att studera rörliga mål: om villkoren för evidens och kunskapsproduktion i socialt arbete. (To study mobile (movable) targets: on the conditions of evidence and knowledge production in social work). *Socialvetenskaplig Tidskrift (Social Science Journal)*, 14(1), 77–82.

Bergmark, A. and Lundström, T. (2002). Education, practice and research: knowledge and attitudes to knowledge of Swedish social workers. *Social Work Education*, 21(3), 359–373.

Bergmark, A. and Lundström, T. (2000). Kunskaper och kunskapssyn: om socialarbetare inom socialtjä¨nsten (Knowledge and views upon knowledge: about social workers within social care). *Socionomens Forskningssupplement*, 12, 1–16.

Bergmark, A. and Lundström, T. (1998). Metoder i socialt arbete (Methods in social work). *Socialvetenskaplig Tidskrift (Social Science Journal)*, 4(5), 291–314.

Bero, L.A., Grilli, R., Grimshaw, J.M., Harvey, E., Oxman, A.D. and Thomson, M. (1998). Closing the gap between research and practice: an overview of systematic reviews of interventions to promote the implementation of research findings. *British Medical Journal*, 317, 465–468.

Besa, D. (1994). Evaluating narrative family therapy using single-system research designs. *Research on Social Work Practice*, 3, 309–325.

Bhaskar, R. (1975). *A realist theory of science*. York: Alma Book Co.

Bilsker, D. and Goldner, E.M. (2000). Teaching evidence based practice in mental health. *Research on Social Work Practice*, 10(5), 664–669.

Bilson, A. (2004). *Evidence-based practice in social work*. London: Whiting & Birch Publishers.

Blau, J.N. (1997). Evidence-based medicine. *Journal of Evaluation in Clinical Practice*, 3(2), 149–151.

Bledsoe, S.E., Weissman, M.M., Mullen, E.J., Ponniah, K., Gameroff, M.J., Verdeli, H., Mufson, L., Fitterling, H. and Wickramaratne, P. (2007). Empirically supported psychotherapy in social work training programs: does the definition of evidence matter? *Research on Social Work Practice*, 17, 449–455.

Bloom, M. and Fischer, J. (1982). *Evaluating practice: guidelines for the accountable professional*. Englewood Cliffs, NJ: Prentice-Hall.

Bloom, M. and Gordon, W.E. (1978). Measurement through practice, *Journal of Education for Social Work*, 14(1), 10–15.

Bloom, M., Fischer, J. and Orme, J. (2003). *Evaluating practice: guidelines for the accountable professional.* Boston: Allyn and Bacon.

Blythe, B.J. and Briar, S. (1985). Developing empirically based models of practice. *Social Work*, 30, 483–488.

Bodenhausen, G.V. and Lichtenstein, M. (1987) Social stereotypes and information-processing strategies: the impact of task complexity. *Journal of Personality and Social Psychology*, 52, 871–880.

Boruch, R. (1994). The future of controlled randomized experiments: a briefing. *Evaluation Practice*, 15(3) 265–274.

Boruch, R., Bullock, M., Cheek, D., Cooper, H., Davies, P., McCord, J., Soydan, H., Thomas, H. and Moya, D. (2001). The Campbell Collaboration: concept, status and plans. *Third International Inter-disciplinary Evidence-Based Policies and Indicator Systems Conference*, CEM Centre, University of Durham. Retrieved 2 September 2008. http://cem.dur.ac.uk

Boruch, R.F., Petrosino, A. and Chalmers, I. (1999). The Campbell Collaboration: a proposal for multinational, continuous and systematic reviews of evidence. In Davies, A., Petrosino, A. and Chalmers, I. (eds). *Proceedings of the International Meeting on Systematic Reviews of the Effects of Social and Educational Interventions July 15–16.* London: University College – London, School of Public Policy.

Boruch, R.F., Soydan, H., de Moya, D. and the Campbell Collaboration Steering Committee (2004). The Campbell Collaboration. *Brief Treatment and Crisis Intervention*, 4, 277–287.

Bowker, G.C. and Leigh Star, S. (1999). *Sorting things out: classification and its consequences* [inside technology]. Cambridge, MA.: MIT Press.

Brekke, J.S. (1986). Scientific imperatives in social work research: pluralism is not scepticism, *Social Service Review*, 60(4), 538–554.

Brekke, J.S., Ell, K. and Palinkas, L.A. (2007). Translational science at the National Institute of Mental Health: can social work take its rightful place? *Research on Social Work Practice*, 17(1), 123–133.

Briar, S. (1973). The age of accountability. *Social Work*, 8, 2–14.

Briggs, D.C. (2004). Causal inference from the Heckman model. *Journal of Educational and Behavioral Statistics*, 29(4), 397–420.

Burkman, E. (1987). Factors affecting utilization. In Gagne, R.M. (ed.). *Instructional technology: foundations*. Hillsdale, NJ: Lawrence Erlbaum.

Burtless, G. (2002). Randomized field trials for policy evaluation. In Mosteller, F. and Boruch, R. (eds). *Evidence matters: randomized trials in education research.* Washington, DC: Brookings Institution Press. 179–197.

Cabinet Office (1999a). *Modernising government.* Presented to Parliament by Command of Her Majesty, 30 March 1999, White Paper. London: HMSO.

Cabinet Office (1999b). *Professional policy making for the twenty-first century.* Report by Strategic Policy Making Team, Cabinet Office, London. Retrieved 23 September 2008. http://www.nationalschool.gov.uk/policyhub/docs/profpolicymaking.pdf

Callon, M. (1991). Techno-economic networks and irreversibility. In Law, J. (ed.). *A sociology of monsters: essays on power, technology and domination.* London: Routledge.

Callon, M. (1986). Some elements of a sociology of translation: domestication of the scallops and the fishermen of St Brieuc Bay. In Law, J. (ed.). *Power, action and belief: a new sociology of knowledge?* London: Routledge.

Callon, M. and Law, J. (1982). On interests and their transformation: enrolment and counter-enrolment. *Social Studies of Science*, 12, 612–625.

Callon, M., Law, J. and Rip, A. (eds). (1986). *Mapping the dynamics of science and technology: sociology of science in the real world*. London: Macmillan.

Campbell Collaboration (nd). *Campbell Library of Systematic Reviews*. Retrieved 7 September 2008. http://www.campbellcollaboration.org/campbell_library/index.php.

Cannella, G.S. and Lincoln, Y.S. (2004). Dangerous discourses II: comprehending and countering the redeployment of discourses (and resources) in the generation of liberatory inquiry. *Qualitative Inquiry*, 10(2), 165–174.

Castells, M. (2002). Materials for an exploratory theory of the network society. *British Journal of Sociology*, 51(1), 5–24.

Centre for Evidence-Based Social Services (CEBSS). Newsletters, Numbers 4–16 published between 1999 and 2004. University of Exeter, Exeter, UK. Retrieved 23 September 2008. http://www.ripfa.org.uk/aboutus/archive/index.asp?TOPcatID=6

Chambless, D.L. (2002). Identification of empirically supported counseling psychology interventions: commentary. *The Counseling Psychologist*, 30, 302–308.

Chambless, D.L., Baker, M.J., Baucom, D.H., Beutler, L.E., Calhoun, K.S., Crits-Christoph, P. *et al*. (1998). Update on empirically validated therapies II. *The Clinical Psychologist*, 15(1), 3–16.

Charlton, B.G. (1997). Restoring the balance: evidence-based medicine put in its place. *Journal of Evaluation in Clinical Practice*, 3(2), 87–98.

Cheetham, J. (1997). Evaluating social work: progress and prospects. *Research on Social Work Practice*, 7(3), 291–310.

Cheetham, J. (1992). Evaluating social work effectiveness. *Research on Social Work Practice*, 2(3), 265–287.

Cheetham, J., Mullen, E.J., Soydan, H. and Tengvald, K. (1998). Evaluation as a tool in the development of social work discourse: national diversity or shared preoccupations? Reflections from a conference. *Evaluation*, 4(1), 9–24.

Chiang, J.H. (1999). Network-based decision making via generalized fuzzy integral operators. *International Journal of Intelligent Systems*, 14(7), 697–716.

Claridge, J.A. and Fabian, T.C. (2005). History and development of evidence-based medicine. *World Journal of Surgery*, 29(5), 547–553.

Clegg, S. (2005). Evidence-based practice in educational research: a critical realist critique of systematic review. *British Journal of Sociology of Education*, 26(3), 415–428.

Closs, S.J. and Lewin, R.J.P. (1998) Perceived barriers to research utilisation: a survey of four therapies. *British Journal of Therapy & Rehabilitation*, 5, 151–155.

Cochrane Collaboration (nd.1). *Product descriptions*. Wiley Interscience. Retrieved 8 September 2008. http://0-www3.interscience.wiley.com.library.newcastle.edu.au/cgi-bin/mrwhome/106568753/ProductDescriptions.html

Cochrane Collaboration (nd.2). *Glossary of Cochrane Collaboration and research terms*. Wiley Interscience. Retrieved 8 September 2008. http://0-www.cochrane.org.library.newcastle.edu.au/resources/glossary.htm

Cochrane Collaboration (nd.3). *Cochrane Qualitative Research Methods Group*. Wiley Interscience. Retrieved 8 September 2008. http://0-www.mrw.interscience.wiley.com.library.newcastle.edu.au/cochrane/clabout/articles/CE000142/frame.html

Cody, N. (1991). The association between client and therapist interpersonal processes and outcomes in psychodynamic psychotherapy. *Research on Social Work Practice*, 1, 122–138.

Cohen, A.M., Stavri, P.Z. and Hersh, W.R. (2004). A categorization and analysis of the criticisms of evidence-based medicine. *International Journal of Medical Information*, 73, 35–43.

Colgan, C. and Cheers, B. (2002). The problem of justification in social work. *Australian Social Work*, 55(2), 109–118.

Cook, T.D. and Payne, M.R. (2002). Objecting to the objections to using random assignment in educational research. In Mosteller, F. and Boruch, R. (eds). *Evidence matters: randomized trials in education research.* Washington, DC: Brookings Institution Press. 150–178.

Coran, E. and Fisher, M. (2006). *The conduct of systematic research reviews for SCIE knowledge reviews.* London: Social Care Institute for Excellence.

Corcoran, K. (2007). From the scientific revolution to evidence-based practice: teaching the short history with a long past. *Research on Social Work Practice*, 17, 548–552.

Corcoran, K. and Fischer, J. (2000a). *Measures for clinical practice. Vol. 1: Couples, families and children.* New York: Free Press.

Corcoran, K. and Fischer, J. (2000b). *Measures for clinical practice. Vol. 2: Adults.* New York: Free Press.

Corcoran, K. and Vandiver, V.L. (2006). Implementing best practice and expert consensus procedures. In Roberts, A.R. and Yeager, K.R. (eds). *Foundations of evidence-based practice.* Oxford: Oxford University Press.

Corrigan, P. and Leonard, P. (1978). *Social work under capitalism.* London: Macmillan.

Cournoyer, B.R. and Powers, G.T. (2002). Evidence-based social work: the quiet revolution continues. In Roberts, A.R. and Greene, G.J. (eds). *Social workers' desk reference.* New York: Oxford University Press. 798–807.

Crawford, C.S. (2004). Actor network theory. In Ritzer, G. (ed.). *Encyclopedia of Social Theory.* London: Sage.

Crisp, B.R. (2004). Evidence based practice and the borders of data in the global information era. *Journal of Social Work Education*, 40, 73–86.

D'Cruz, H., Gillingham, P. and Melendez, S. (2007). Reflexivity, its meanings and relevance for social work: a critical review of the literature. *British Journal of Social Work*, 37(1), 73–90.

Dasari, B.D. (2003). Why occupational therapy needs evidence based practice. Paper presented at the *3rd Asia Pacific Occupational Therapy Congress*, Singapore, 15–18 September 2003.

Daukas, N. (2006). Epistemic trust and social location. *Episteme: A Journal of Social Epistemology*, 3(1), 109–124.

Davenport, T.H. and Prusak, L. (1998). *Working knowledge: how organizations manage what they know.* Boston: Harvard Business School Press.

Davies, A.R. (2002). Power, politics and networks: shaping partnerships for sustainable communities. *Area*, 34(2), 190–203.

De La Parra, G. and Del Rio, M. (2005). Can psychoanalysis and systemic research work productively together? *International Journal of Psychoanalysis*, 86, 151–154.

Denvall, V. (2008). Evidence in action: a Thompsonian perspective on evidence-based decision-making in social work. *European Journal of Social Work*, 11(1), 29–42.

Denzin, N.K. and Lincoln, Y.S. (eds). (1994). *Handbook of qualitative research.* Thousand Oaks, CA: Sage Publications.

Denzin, N.K., Lincoln, Y.S. and Smith, L.T. (2008). *Handbook of critical and Indigenous methodologies.* New York: Sage.

Dore, I.J. (2006). Evidence focused social care: on target or off-side? *Social Work & Society*, 4(2). Available online at http://www.socwork.net/2006/2/articles/dore

Drisko, J.W. (2004). Common factors in psychotherapy outcome: meta-analytic findings and their implications for practice and research. *Families in Society*, 85(1), 81–90.

Echholm, M. (2004). *Evidence-based policy research: some Swedish lessons*. Paper presented at the *First OECD Conference on Evidence Based Policy Research*, 19–20 April, Washington. Retrieved 12 September 2008. Available online at http://www. excelgov.org/usermedia/images/uploads/PDFs/OECD-Ekholm.pdf

Ekbia, H.R. and Hara, N. (2008). The quality of evidence in knowledge management research: practitioner versus scholarly literature. *Journal of Information Science*, 34(1), 10–126.

Elliott, J. (2001). Making evidence-based practice educational. *British Educational Research Journal*, 27(5), 555–574.

English, B., Gaha, J. and Gibbons, J. (1994). Preparing social workers for an uncertain future. In Chen, S.E., Cowdroy, R., Kingsland, A. and Ostwald, M. (eds). *Reflections on problem based learning*. Sydney: Wild and Woolley.

Epstein, I. (1996). In quest of a research-based model for clinical practice: or, why can't a social worker be more like a researcher? *Social Work Research*, 20(2), 97–100.

Erle, J.B. and Goldberg, D.A. (2003). The course of 253 analyses from selection to outcome. *Journal of the American Psychoanalytic Association*, 51, 257–292.

Evidence-based Medicine Working Group (1992). Evidence-based medicine: a new approach to teaching the practice of medicine. *JAMA*, 268, 2420–2425.

Eysenck, H.J. (1952). The effect of psychotherapy: an evaluation. *Journal of Consulting Psychology*, 16, 319–324.

Fairbanks, R.P., II. (2008) *How it works: post-welfare politics in the Kensington recovery house movement*. Chicago: The University of Chicago Press.

Farrel, L., Cunningham, M., Haigh, V., Irozuru, E. and Roberts Cuffin, T. (1999). Virtual evidence: helping primary care practitioners access and implement evidence-based information. *Health Informatics Journal*, 5(4), 188–192.

Fauth, R. and Mahdon, M. (2007). Improving social and health care services. *SCIE Knowledge Review 16*. London: Social Care Institute of Excellence.

Fawcett, B. and Featherstone, B. (1998). Quality assurance and evaluation in social work in a postmodern era. In Carter, J. (ed.). *Postmodernity and the fragmentation of welfare*. London: Routledge.

Fawcett, B., Featherstone, B., Fook, J. and Rossiter, A. (2000). (eds). *Research and practice in social work: postmodern feminist perspectives*. London: Routledge.

Fawcett, B. (2008). Postmodernism. In Gray, M. and Webb, S.A. (eds). *Social work theories and methods*. London: Sage, 119–128.

Fejo-King, C. (2005). Decolonising research from an Australian indigenous research perspective. *The National Coalition of Aboriginal and Torres Strait Islander Social Workers Association E-Journal*. Available online at: http://trabajosocialalternativo. googlepages.com/Decolonising20Research20from20and20Australian20Indigenous20 Perspective.pdf. Retrieved 9 January 2009.

Ferguson, H. (2003). Outline of a critical best practice perspective on social work and social care. *British Journal of Social Work*, 1005–1024.

Field, M.J. and Lohr, K.N. (eds). (1990). *Clinical Practice Guidelines: directions for a new program*. Institute of Medicine, Washington, DC: National Academy Press.

Fielding, N. and Fielding, J. (1986). *Linking data: the articulation of qualitative and quantitative methods in social research*. London: Sage.

Fischer, J. (2009). *Toward evidence-based practice: variations on a theme*. Chicago: Lyceum.

Fischer, J. (2004). Reflections on destroying social work. *Reflections: Narratives of Professional Helping*, 10.

Fischer, J. (1993). Empirically-based practice: the end of ideology? *Journal of Social Service Research*, 15, 19–64.

Fischer, J. (1981). The social work revolution. *Social Work*, 26, 199–209.

Fischer, J. (1978a). Does anything work? *Journal of Social Service Research*, 1, 215–243.

Fischer, J. (1978b). *Effective casework practice: an eclectic approach*. New York: McGraw-Hill.

Fischer, J. (1976). *The effectiveness of social casework*. Springfield, IL: Charles C. Thomas.

Fischer, J. (1973a). Is casework effective? A review. *Social Work*, 18, 5–21.

Fischer, J. (1973b). Interpersonal helping: emerging approaches for social work practice. Springfield, IL: Charles C. Thomas.

Fischer, J. (1973c). Has mighty casework struck out? *Social Work*, 18, 107–110.

Fonagy, E. (ed.). (2002). An open door review of outcome studies in psychoanalysis (2nd edn). London: International Psychoanalytic Association.

Fook, J. (2002). *Social work: critical theory and practice*. London: Sage.

Fook, J. (1993). *Radical casework: a theory of practice*. St Leonards: Allen and Unwin.

Fuller, S. (1993). Disciplinary boundaries and the rhetoric of social sciences. In Messer-Davidow, E., Shumway, D. and Sylvan, D.J. (eds). *Knowledges: historical and critical studies in disciplinarity*. Virginia: University of Virginia Press.

Freemantle, N., Harvey, E.L., Wolf, F., Grimshaw, J.M., Grilli, R. and Bero, L.A. (2001). Printed educational materials: Effects on professional practice and health care outcomes. *Cochrane Database Systematic Rev*, (2), CD000172.

Gadamer, H-G. (1989). *Truth and method*. New York: Crossroad.

Gale, A.W. (1998). Evidence-based practice: MIDCAB or MADCAB. *Asian Cardiovascular and Thoracic Annals*, 6, 243–244.

Gambrill, E. (2007). Transparency as the route to evidence-informed professional education. *Research on Social Work Practice*, 17(5), 553–560.

Gambrill, E. (2006a). *Social work practice: a critical thinker's guide*. Oxford: Oxford University Press.

Gambrill, E. (2006b). Evidence-based practice and policy: choices ahead. *Research on Social Work Practice*, 16(3), 338–357.

Gambrill, E. (2005). *Critical thinking in clinical practice: improving the quality of judgments and decisions* (2nd edn). New Jersey: John Wiley and Sons.

Gambrill, E. (2003). Evidence-based practice: sea change or the emperor's new clothes? *Journal of Social Work Education*, 39, 3–23.

Gambrill, E. (1983). *Casework: a competency-based approach*. Englewood Cliffs, NJ: Prentice-Hall.

Gambrill, E.D. (2004). The future of evidence-based social work practice. In Thyer, B.A. and Kazi, M.A.F. (eds). *International perspectives on evidence-based practice in social work*. Birmingham: Venture Press.

Gambrill, E.D. (2001). Social work: an authority-based profession. *Research on Social Work Practice*, 11(2), 166–175.

Gambrill, E.D. (1999). Evidence-based practice: an alternative to authority-based practice. *Families in Society: The Journal of Contemporary Human Services*, 80(4), 341–350.

Garretsen, H., Bongers, I. and Rodenburg, G. (2005). Evidence-based work in the Dutch welfare sector. *British Journal of Social Work*, 655–665.

Germain, C. (1981). The ecological approach to people–environmental transactions. *Social Casework*, 62(6), 323–331.

Germain, C. and Gitterman, A. (1980). *The life model of social work practice*. New York: Columbia University Press.

Gibbons, J. (2001). Effective practice: social work's long history of concern about outcomes. *Australian Social Work*, 54(3), 3–13.

Gibbons, J. and Gray, M. (2005). Teaching social work students about social policy. *Australian Social Work*, 58(1), 58–75.

Gibbons, J. and Gray, M. (2004). Critical thinking as integral to social work practice. *Journal of Teaching in Social Work*, 24(1/2), 19–38.

Gibbons, J. and Gray, M. (2002). An integrated and experience-based approach to social work education: the Newcastle model. *Journal of Social Work Education*, 21(5), 529–549.

Gibbons, M. (2000). Mode 2 society and the emergence of context-sensitive science. *Science and Public Policy*, 26(5): 159–163.

Gibbons, M., Limoges, C., Nowotny, H., Schwartzman, S., Scott, P. and Trow, M. (1994). *The new production of knowledge: the dynamics of science and research in contemporary societies*. London: Sage.

Gibbs, A. (2001). The changing nature and context of social work research. *British Journal of Social Work*, 31, 687–704.

Gibbs, L. (2003). *Evidence-based practice for the helping professions*. Pacific Grove, CA: Brooks/Cole.

Gibbs, L. and Gambrill, E. (2002). Evidence-based practice: counterarguments to objections. *Research on Social Work Practice*, 12(3), 452–476.

Giddens, A. (1976). *New rules of sociological method*. New York: Basic Books.

Gilgun, J.F. (2005). The four cornerstones of evidence-based practice in social work. *Research on Social Work Practice*, 15(1), 52–61.

Gira, E.C., Kessler, M.L. and Poertner, J. (2004). Influencing social workers to use research evidence in practice: lessons from medicine, allied health professions. *Research on Social Work Practice*, 14(2), 68–79.

Glisson, C. and Fischer, J. (1986). Statistical training for social workers. *Journal of Social Work Education*, 23(2), 50–58.

Goldstein, H. (2001). *Experiential learning: a foundation for social work education and practice*. Washington, DC: Council of Social Work Education.

Goldstein, H. (1992). If social work hasn't made progress as a science, might it be an art? *Families in Society*, 73(1), 48–55.

Goldstein, H. (1991). Qualitative research and social work practice: partners in discovery. *Journal of Sociology and Social Welfare*, 18(4), 101–119.

Goldstein, H. (1988). Humanistic alternatives to the limits of scientific knowledge. *Social Thought*, 19(1), 181–187.

Goldstein, H. (1987). The neglected moral link in social work practice. *Social Work*, 32(3), 181–187.

Goldstein, H. (1973). *Social work practice: a unitary approach*. Columbia, South Carolina: University of South Carolina Press.

Gould, N. and Kendall, T. (2007). Developing NICE/SCIE guidelines for dementia care: the challenges of enhancing the evidence base for social health care. *British Journal of Social Work*, 37, 475–490.

Gould, N. and Taylor, I. (eds). (1996). *Reflective learning for social work: research, theory and practice*. Aldershot, Hants: Arena.

Gray, M. (2008). Some considerations on the debate on social work in China: who speaks for whom? *International Journal of Social Welfare*, 17(4), 400–406.

Gray, M. (2007). The not so critical 'critical reflection'. Editorial, *Australian Social Work*, 60(2), 131–135.

Gray, M. (2005). Dilemmas of international social work: paradoxical processes in indigenisation, imperialism and universalism. *International Journal of Social Welfare*, 14(2), 230–237.

Gray, M. and Gibbons, J. (2007). There are no answers, only choices: teaching ethical decision making in social work. *Australian Social Work*, 60(2), 222–238.

Gray, M. and Gibbons, J. (2002). Experience-based learning and its relevance to social work practice. *Australian Social Work*, 55(4), 279–291.

Gray, M. and Lovat, T. (2006). The shaky high moral ground of postmodern 'ethics'. *Social Work/Maatskaplike*, 42, 201–212.

Gray, M. and McDonald, C. (2006). Pursuing good practice? The limits of evidence-based practice. *Journal of Social Work*, 1, 7–20.

Gray, M. and Webb, S.A. (eds). (2008). *Social work theories and methods*. London: Sage.

Gray, M., Coates, J. and Yellow Bird, M. (eds). (2008). *Indigenous social work around the world: towards culturally relevant education and practice*. Aldershot, Hants: Ashgate.

Graybeal, C.T. (2007). Evidence for the art of social work. *Families in Society*, 88(4), 513–523.

Greenhalgh, T. (2001) *How to read a paper: the basics of evidence-based medicine*. Wiley Blackwell: Oxford.

Grinnell, R.M. Jnr (1988). *Social work research and evaluation*. Itasca, Illinois: F.E. Peacock Publishers.

Grint, K. and Woolgar, S. (1997). *The machine at work: technology, work and society*. Cambridge: Polity Press.

Guardian (2007). *Interview with Julie Jones: 'The Rule of Evidence'*. Interviewed by David Brindle, Wednesday, 28 March, p. 5. Retrieved 3 October 2008. http://www.guardian. co.uk/society/2007/mar/28/socialcare.guardiansocietysupplement

Gueron, J.M. (2007). Building evidence: what it takes and what it yields. *Research on Social Work Practice*, 17(1), 134–142.

Gueron, J.M. (2002). The politics of random assignment: implementing studies and affecting policy. In Mosteller, F. and Boruch, R. (eds). *Evidence matters: randomized trials in education research*. Washington, DC: Brookings Institution Press. 15–49.

Gustle, L.-H., Hansson, K., Lundh, L.-G. and Lofholm, C.A. (2007). Blueprints in Sweden. Symptom load in Swedish adolescents in studies of functional family therapy (FFT), multisystemic therapy (MST) and multidimensional treatment foster care (MTFC). *Nordic Journal of Psychiatry*, 61(6), 443–451.

Gustle, L.-H., Hansson, K., Sundell, K. and Lofholm, C.A. (2008). Implementation of evidence-based models in social work practice: practitioners' perspectives on an MST trial in Sweden. *Journal of Child and Adolescent Substance Abuse*, 17(3), 111–125.

Habermas, J. (1968). *Knowledge and human interests*. Cambridge: Polity Press.

Hall, J.C. (2008). A practitioner's application and deconstruction of evidence-based practice. *Families in Society: The Journal of Contemporary Social Services*, 89(3), 385–393.

Hammersley, M. (2003). Social research today: some dilemmas and distinctions. *Qualitative Social Work*, 2(1), 25–44.

Hammersley, M. (2002) *Educational research, policymaking and practice*. London: Paul Chapman.

Hammersley, M. (2001). On 'systematic' reviews of research literature: a 'narrative' response to Evans and Benefield. *British Educational Research Journal*, 27(5), 543–554.

Hampshire Social Services (1999). *Evidence-based practice in Hampshire Social Services: notes on our strategy*. Hampshire, UK: Hampshire Social Services.

Harries, U., Elliot, H. and Higgins, A. (1999). Evidence-based policy-making in the NHS: exploring the interface between research and the commissioning process. *Journal of Public Health Medicine*, 21(1), 29–36.

Hausman, A.J. (2002). Implications of evidence-based practice for community health. *American Journal of Community Psychology*, 30(3), 149–166.

Heineman Pieper, M. (1989). The heuristic paradigm: a unifying and comprehensive approach to social work research. *Smith College Studies*, 60(1), 8–34.

Heineman Pieper, M. (1981). The obsolete scientific imperative in social work research and practice. *Social Service Review*, 55(3), 371–397.

Hill, H.C. (2003). Understanding implementation: street-level bureaucrats' resources for reform. *Journal of Public Administration Research and Theory*, 13(3), 265–283.

Hodson, R. (2003). *Leading the drive for evidence based practice in services for children and families: summary report of a study conducted for research in practice*. UK: Research in Practice.

Holosko, M.J. (2004). Evidence-based practice in Canada. In Thyer, B.A. and Kazi, M.A.F. (eds). (2004). *International perspectives on evidence-based practice in social work*. Birmingham, UK: Venture Press. 149–166.

House of Commons Science and Technology Select Committee (2007). Appendix to the Select Committee Report. Retrieved 23 September 2008. http://www.parliament.the-stationery-office.co.uk/pa/cm200607/cmselect/cmsctech/307/30704.htm

House of Commons Science and Technology Select Committee (2006). *Scientific advice, risk and evidence in policy making*, Seventh Report, HMSO, London. Retrieved 23 September 2008. http://www.publications.parliament.uk/pa/cm200506/cmselect/cmsctech/900/90002.htm#evidence

Howard, M.O. and Jensen, J.M. (1999). Clinical practice guidelines: should social work develop them? *Research on Social Work Practice*, 9, 283–301.

Howard, M.O., Allen-Meares, P. and Ruffolo, M.C. (2007). Teaching evidence-based practice: strategic and pedagogical recommendations for schools of social work. *Research on Social Work Practice*, 17, 561–568.

Howard, M.O., McMillen, C.J. and Pollio, D.E. (2003). Teaching evidence-based practice: toward a new paradigm for social work education. *Research on Social Work Practice*, 13(2), 234–259.

Howe, K. (2004). A critique of experimentalism. *Qualitative Inquiry*, 10(1), 42–61.

Hudson, B. and Macdonald, G. (1986). *Behavioural social work*. London: Macmillan.

Hudson, W.W. (1982a). *The clinical measurement package: a field manual*. Homewood, Ill.: Dorsey Press.

Hudson, W.W. (1982b). Scientific imperatives in social work research and practice. *Social Service Review*, 56(2), 242–258.

Hurwitz, B. (2004). How does evidence based guidance influence determinations of medical negligence? *British Medical Journal*, 329, 1024–1028.

Hustler, D. and Stronach, I. (2001). Old whine in new battles. Editorial. *British Educational Research Journal*, 27(5), 523–525.

Hyams, A.L., Brandenburg, J.A., Lipsitz, S.R., Shapiro, D.W. and Brennan, T.A. (1995). Practice guidelines and malpractice litigation: a two way street. *Annals of Internal Medicine*, 22, 450–455.

Imre, R.W. (1984). The nature of knowledge in social work. *Social Work*, 29(1), 41–45.

Independent Review Group (1994). *A wider strategy for research and development relating to the personal social service*. Report to the Director of Research and Development, Department of Health, by an independent review group (chaired by Gilbert Smith). London: The Stationery Office.

Ixer, G. (1999). There's no such thing as reflection. *British Journal of Social Work*, 29(4), 513–527.

Jayaratne, S. and Levy, R.L. (1979). *Empirical clinical practice*. New York: Columbia University.

Johnson-Woods, T. (2002). *Big Brother.* St Lucia: Queensland. 30–131.

Jones, M. (1990). Understanding social work: a matter of interpretation? *British Journal of Social Work*, 20(3), 184–196.

Kahneman, D. and Tversky, A. (1973). On the psychology of prediction. *Psychological Review*, 80, 237–251.

Kahneman, D., Slovic, P. and Tversky, A. (1982). *Judgement under uncertainty: heuristics and biases*. Cambridge University Press, Cambridge.

Kärrholm, M. (2007). The materiality of territorial production: a conceptual discussion of territoriality, materiality, and the everyday life of public space. *Space and Culture*, 10, 437–453.

Karvinen, S. (1999). Sosiaalityön tutkimuksen jännitekenttä, *Janus*, 4, 397–386.

Karvinen, S. (1996). *Sosiaalityön ammatillisuus modernista professiuonaalisuudesta reflektiiviseen asiantuntijuuteen* (The idea of professional method and reflective practice in social work from modern professionalism to new expertise). Kuopio, Kuopion yliopiston julkaisuja E Yhteiskuntatieteet.

Karvinen, S., Pösö, T. and Satka, M. (eds). (1999). *Reconstructing social work research*. Jyväskylä: University of Jyväskylä SoPhi.

Kazi, M.A.F. and Wilson, J. (1996). Applying single-case evaluation in social work. *British Journal of Social Work*, 26, 699–717.

Kindler, H. (2008). Developing evidence-based child protection practice: a view from Germany. *Research on Social Work Practice*, 18(4), 319–324.

Kindler, H., Lilliog, S., Blüml, H., Meysen, T. and Werner, A. (2006). *Child endangerment according to § 1666 civil code and child protection service*. Munich, Germany: DJI. Available online at: http://www.dji.de/asd

Kirk, S.A. (1999). Good intentions are not enough: practice guidelines for social work. *Research on Social Work Practice*, 9(3), 302–310.

Kondrat, M.E. (1992). Reclaiming the practical: formal and substantive rationality in social work practice. *Social Service Review*, 66(2), 237–255.

Korn, E.L. (2006). Comment: causal inference in the medical area. *Statistical Science*, 21(3), 310–312.

Latour, B. (2002). Morality and technology: the ends and the means. *Theory, Culture & Society*, 19(5/6), 247–260.

Latour, B. (1999). *Pandora's hope: essays on the reality of science studies*. Cambridge MA.: Harvard University Press.

Latour, B. (1996) *Aramis, or the love of technology*. Cambridge MA.: Harvard University Press.

Latour, B. (1988). *The pasteurization of France*. Cambridge, MA: Harvard University Press.

Latour, B. (1987). *Science in action*. MA: Harvard University Press.

Latour, B. and Woolgar, S. (1991). *Laboratory life: the construction of scientific fact* (3rd edn). London: Sage.

Lave, J. and Wenger, E. (1991). *Situated learning: legitimate peripheral participation.* Cambridge: Cambridge University Press.

Law, J. (1999a). After ANT: complexity, naming and topology. In Hassard, J. (ed.). *Actor network theory and after.* Oxford: Blackwell/*The Sociological Review.*

Law, J. (1999b) Introduction. In Law, J. and Hassard, J. (eds). *Actor-network theory and after.* Oxford: Blackwell. 1–14.

Law, J. (1992). Note on the theory of actor-network: ordering, strategy and heterogeneity. *Systems Practice*, 5, 379–393.

Law, J. and Hassard, J. (eds). (1999). *Actor network theory and after.* Oxford: Blackwell.

Leach, M. (2006). Evidence-based practice: a framework for clinical practice and research design. *International Journal of Nursing Practice*, 12(5), 248–251.

Lee, A. (1999). Researching MIS. In Currie, W. and Galliers, B. (eds). *Rethinking management information systems: an interdisciplinary perspective.* Oxford: Oxford University Press. 7–27.

Lee, N. and Hassard, J. (1999) Organization unbound: actor-network theory, research strategy and institutional flexibility. *Organization* 6(3), 391–404.

Leung, G.M. (2001). Evidence-based practice revisited. *Asia Pacific Journal of Public Health*, 13, 116–121.

Lewis, R.A., Urquhart, C.J. and Rolinson, J. (1998). Health professionals' attitudes towards evidence-based medicine and the role of the information professional in exploitation of the research evidence. *Journal of Information Science*, 24, 281–290.

Liel, C. and Kindler, H. (2006). *Analysis of empirical articles in five volumes of German social work journals.* Munich, Germany: DJI.

Lincoln, Y.S. and Cannella, G. (2004). Dangerous discourses: methodological conservatism and governmental regimes of truth. *Qualitative Inquiry*, 10, 5–14.

Lincoln, Y.S. and Guba, E.G. (1985). *Naturalistic inquiry.* Beverly Hills, CA: Sage.

Lindsey, D. and Shlonsky, A. (eds). (2008). *Child welfare research: advances for practice and policy.* New York: Oxford University Press.

Lipsey, M.W. (2009). The primary factors that characterise effective interventions with juvenile offenders: a meta-analytic overview. *Victims and Offenders* (in press).

Lipsey, M.W. (2003). Those confounded moderators in meta-analysis: good, bad and ugly. *The Annals of the American Academy of Political and Social Science*, 589, 69–81.

Lipsey, M.W. and Wilson, D.B. (2000). *Practical meta-analysis.* London: Sage.

Littell, J. (2008). How do we know what works? The quality of published reviews of evidence-based practices. In Lindsey, D. and Shlonsky, A. (eds). (2008). *Child welfare research: advances for practice and policy.* New York: Oxford University Press.

Littell, J. (2005). Lessons from a systematic review of effects of multisystemic therapy. *Children and Youth Services Review*, 27(4), 445–463.

Littell, J., Corcoran, J. and Pillai, V. (2008). *Systematic reviews and meta-analysis.* Oxford: Oxford University Press.

Lovelock, R., Hamilton, K.M. and Powell, J. (2004). *Reflecting on social work: discipline and profession.* Aldershot, Hants: Ashgate.

Lucas, A.M. (2008). Evidence-based practice and the de-professionalization of practitioners. *Studies in Science Education*, 44(10), 83–92.

Luckock, B., Lefevre, M., Orr, D., Jones, M., Marchant, R. and Tanner, K. (2006) Teaching, learning and assessing communication skills with children and young people in social work education. *SCIE Knowledge Review 12.* London: Social Care Institute of Excellence.

McBeath, G. and Webb, S.A. (1991). Social work, modernity and post modernity. *Sociological Review*, 39(4), 745–762.

McCarthy, A. and Martin-McDonald, K. (2007). 'A politics of what': the enactment of peritoneal dialysis in indigenous Australians. *Sociology of Health & Illness*, 29(1), 82–99.

McCracken, S.G. and Marsh, J.C. (2008). Practitioner expertise in evidence-based practice decision making. *Research on Social Work Practice*, 18(4), 301–310.

Macdonald, G. (2004). Intervening with neglect. In Taylor, J. and Daniel, B. (eds). *Neglect: issues for health and social care*. London: Jessica Kingsley.

Macdonald, G. (2003a). *Effective interventions for child abuse and neglect: an evidence-based approach to planning and evaluating interventions*. Chichester: Wiley.

Macdonald, G. (2003b). *Using systematic reviews to improve social care*. London: Social Care Institute for Excellence.

Macdonald, G. (2001). *Effective interventions for child abuse and neglect: an evidence-based approach to planning and evaluating interventions*. Chichester: Wiley.

Macdonald, G. (1999a). Evidence-based social care: wheels off the runway? *Public Money & Management*, 19(1), 25–32.

Macdonald, G. (1999b). Social work and its evaluation: a methodological dilemma. In Williams, F., Popay, J. and Oakley, A. (eds). *Welfare research: a critical review*. London: Routledge. Available online at: http://www. cambellcollaboration.org/papers/4_progress.pdf

Macdonald. (1999c). 'Systematic review of the effects of day care for pre-school children'. Paper presented as part of a Campbell Collaboration meeting, University College: London, 15–16.

Macdonald, G. (1994). Developing empirically-based practice in probation. *British Journal of Social Work*, 24(4), 405–427.

Macdonald, G. and Roberts, H. (1995). *What works in the early years? Effective interventions for children and their families in health, social welfare, education and child protection*. Essex: Barnardos.

Macdonald, G. and Sheldon, B. with Gillespie, J. (1992). Contemporary studies of the effectiveness of social work. *British Journal of Social Work*, 22(6), 615–643.

Macdonald, G., Higgens, J.P.T. and Ramchandani, P. (2006). Cognitive-behavioural interventions for children who have been sexually abused. *Cochrane Database of Systematic Reviews*, Issue 4, Art. No. CD001930. DOI: 10.1002/14651858.CD001930. pub.2

Machlup, F. (1983). Semantic quirks in studies of information. In Machlup, F. and Mansfield, U. (eds). *The study of information: interdisciplinary messages*. New York, NY: Wiley.

MacKenzie, D. (1996). *Knowing machines: essays on technical change*. Cambridge, MA: MIT Press.

McNeece, C.A. and Thyer, B.A. (2004). Evidence-based practice and social work. *Journal of Evidence-Based Social Work*, 1(1), 7–25.

McWilliam, C.L. (2007). Continuing education at the cutting edge: promoting transformative knowledge translation. *Journal of Continuing Education in the Health Professions*, 27(2), 72–79.

Magill, M. (2006). The future of evidence in evidence-based practice: who will answer the call for clinical relevance? *Journal of Social Work*, 6, 101–115.

Malterud, K. (2001). The art and science of clinical knowledge: evidence beyond measures and numbers. *The Lancet*, 358, 397–400.

Marchant, R., Lefevre, M., Jones, M. and Luckock, B. (2007). Necessary stuff: the social care needs of children with complex health care needs and their families. *SCIE Knowledge Review 18*. London: Social Care Institute of Excellence.

Marsh, P. and Fisher, M. (2005). *Developing the evidence-based for social work and social care practice, Report 10.* London: Social Care Institute of Excellence.

Marthinsen, E. (2004). A mind for learning: merging education, practice and research in social work. *Social Work & Social Sciences Review*, 11(2), 54–66.

Martis, R., Ho, J.J. and Crowther, C.A. (2008). Survey of knowledge and perception on the access to evidence-based practice and clinical practice change among maternal and infant health practitioners in South East Asia. *BMC Pregnancy and Childbirth*, 8:34. DOI:10.1186/1471-2393-8-34. Retrieved 10 September 2008. http://www.biomedcentral.com/1471-2393/8/34

Mattaini, M.A. (1996). The abuse and neglect of single-case designs. *Research on Social Work Practice*, 6(1), 83–90.

Maxwell, J.A. (2004). Reemergent scientism, postmodernism, and dialogue across differences. *Qualitative Inquiry*, 10(1), 35–41.

Merritt, T.A., Gold, M. and Holland, J. (1999). A critical evaluation of clinical practice guidelines in neonatal medicine: does their use improve quality and lower costs? *Journal of Evaluation in Clinical Practice*, 5(2), 169–177.

Messer-Davidow, E., Shumway, D., and Sylvan, D.J. (eds). (1993). *Knowledges: historical and critical studies in disciplinarity.* Virginia: University of Virginia Press.

Meyer, C. (ed.) (1983). *Clinical social work in the ecosystems perspective.* New York: Columbia University Press.

Morago, P. (2006). Evidence-based practice: from medicine to social work. *European Journal of Social Work*, 9(4), 461–477.

Morgan, W.K.C. (1997). On evidence, embellishment and efficacy. *Journal of Evaluation in Clinical Practice*, 3(2), 117–122.

Morse, J.M. (2006). The politics of evidence. *Qualitative Health Research*, 16(3), 395–404.

Mullaly, R. (2007). *The new structural social work.* Don Mills, Ontario: Oxford University Press.

Mullen, E.J. (2006). Choosing outcome measures in systematic reviews: critical challenges. *Research on Social Work Practice*, 16(1), 84–90.

Mullen, E.J. (2002). Evidence-based social work theory and practice: historical and reflective perspective. *4th International Conference on Evaluation for Practice*, University of Tampere, Finland, 4–6 July.

Mullen, E.J. and Bacon, W. (2006). Implementation of practice guidelines and evidence-based treatment: a survey of psychiatrists, psychologists and social workers. In Roberts, A.R. and Yeager, K.R. (eds). *Foundations of evidence-based social work practice.* New York: Oxford University Press.

Mullen, E.J. and Bacon, W. (2004). A survey of practitioner adoption and implementation of practice guidelines and evidence based treatments. In Roberts, A.R. and Yeager, K. (eds). *Evidence based practice manual: research and outcome measures in health and human services*, New York, NY: Oxford University Press. 210–218.

Mullen, E.J. and Bacon, W.F. (2003). Practitioner adoption and implementation of evidence-based effective treatments and issues of quality control. In Rosen, A. and Proctor, E.K. (eds). *Developing practice guidelines for social work intervention: issues, methods, and a research agenda.* Columbia: Columbia University Press.

Mullen, E.J., Bellamy, J.L. and Bledsoe, S.E. (2005). Implementing evidence-based social work practice. In Sommerfeld, P. (ed.). *Evidence-based social work: towards a new professionalism?* New York: Peter Lang Publishing Group.

Mullen, E.J., Bellamy, J.L., Bledsoe, S.E. and Francois, J.J. (2007). Teaching evidence-based practice. *Research on Social Work Practice*, 17(5), 574–582.

Mullen, E.J., Bledsoe, S.E. and Bellamy, J.L. (2008). Implementing evidence-based social work practice. *Research on Social Work Practice*, 18(1), 325–338.

Mullen, E.J., Dumpson, J. *et al.* (1972). *Evaluation of social interventions*. San Francisco: Jossey-Bass.

Mullen, E.J., Shlonsky, A., Bledsoe, S. and Bellamy, J.L. (2005). From concept to implementation: challenges facing evidence-based social work. *Evidence & Policy*, 1, 61–84.

Murdoch, J. (1998) The spaces of actor-network theory. *Geoforum* 29(4), 357–374.

Murphy, A. and McDonald, J. (2004). Power, status and marginalisation: rural social workers and evidence-based practice in multi-disciplinary teams. *Australian Social Work*, 57(2), 127–136.

Murray, S.J., Holmes, D. and Rail, G. (2008). On the constitution and status of 'evidence' in the health sciences. *Journal of Research in Nursing*, 13, 272–280.

Nathan, P. and Gorman, J. (eds). (2007). *A guide to treatments that work*. New York: Oxford University Press.

National Institute for Clinical Excellence (NICE) (2007). NICE guidelines. Retrieved 31 July 2007. http://0-www.nice.org.uk.library.newcastle.edu.au/page.aspx?o=137

National Institute of Mental Health, National Advisory Mental Health Council Behavioral Science Workgroup (2000). *Translating behavioral science into action* (No. NIH 00-4699). Bethesda, MD: National Institute of Mental Health.

National Research Council (2002). *Scientific research in education* (Committee on Scientific Principles for Educational Research, R.J. Shavelson and L. Towne (eds). Center for Education, Division of Behavioral and Social Sciences and Education). Washington, DC: National Academy Press.

Nelson, J.C. (1988). Single-subject research. In Grinnell, R.M. Jnr (ed.). *Social work research and evaluation*. Itasca, Illinois: F.E. Peacock Publishers. 362–399.

New Freedom Commission on Mental Health. (2003). *Achieving the promise: transforming mental health care in America. Final report* (DHHS Publication No. SMA-03-3832). Rockville, MD: United States Department of Health and Human Services. Retrieved 10 August 2008. http://www.mentalhealthcommission.gov/reports/FinalReport/downloads/downloads.html

New York State Office of Mental Health (2001). *Winds of change: creating an environment of quality*. Albany: New York State Office of Mental Health.

Newman, T. (1999). *Evidence-based child care practice*. London, UK: National Children's Bureau. Highlight no. 170.

Newman, T. and McNeish, D. (2005). Promoting evidence based practice in a child care charity: the Barnardo's experience. In Bilson, A. (ed.). *Evidence-based practice in social work*. London: Whiting and Birch.

Newman, T., Moseley, A., Tierney, S. and Ellis, A. (2005). *Evidence-based social work: a guide for the perplexed*. Lyme Regis: Russell House Publishing.

Neyland, D. (2006) Dismissed content and discontent: an analysis of the strategic aspects of actor-network theory. *Science, Technology, and Human Values*, 3, 29–51.

Nisbett, R.E. and Ross, L. (1980). *Human inference: strategies and shortcomings of social judgement*. Englewood Cliffs, NJ: Prentice Hall.

No Child Left Behind Act of 2001, Pub. L. No. 107–110, 115 Stat. 1425 (2002). Retrieved 10 August 2008. http://www.ed.gov/policy/elsec/leg/esea02/107-110.pdf

Oakley, A. (1999) 'Infrastructure for assessing social and educational interventions: the same or different?'. Paper presented at the Campbell Collaboration meeting, University College, London, 15–16 July. Available online at: http://www.ucl.ac.uk/spp/download/publications/SPP-FIN.pdf

Ogden, T. (2008). 'Linking research, policy and practice in Norway: improving the use of evidence in the policy process'. Presentation at the NORFACE seminar, Oslo, 13 October 2008.

Ogden, T. and Hagen, K.A. (2006). Multisystemic therapy of serious behavior problems in youth: sustainability of therapy effectiveness two years after intake. *Child and Adolescent Mental Health*, 11(3), 142–149.

Ogden, T. and Halliday-Boykins, C.A. (2004). Multisystemic treatment of antisocial adolescents in Norway: replication of clinical outcomes outside of the US. *Child and Adolescent Mental Health*, 9(2), 77–83.

Ogden, T., Christensen, B., Sheidow, A.J. and Holth, P. (2008). Bridging the gap between science and practice: the effective nationwide transport of MST programs in Norway. *Journal of Child and Adolescent Substance Abuse*, 17(3), 93–109.

Ogden, T., Hagen, K.A. and Anderson, O. (2007). Sustainability of the effectiveness of a programme of multisystemic treatment (MST) across participant groups in the second year of operation. *Journal of Children's Services*, 2(3), 4–14.

O'Toole, L.J. (1986). Policy recommendations for multi-actor implementation: an assessment of the field. *Journal of Public Policy*, 6(2), 181–210.

Otto, H.-U. and Ziegler, H. (2008). The notion of causal impact in evidence-based social work: an introduction to the special issue on *What Works? Research on Social Work Practice*, 18(4), 273–277.

Owen, M. and Jenson, J.M. (1999). Clinical practice guidelines: should social work develop them? *Research on Social Work Practice*, 9(3), 283–301.

Oxman, A.D. *et al.* (1994). Users' guides to the medical literature, VI. How to use an overview. *JAMA*, 272(17), 1367–1371.

Padgett, D.K. (2005). The *Society for Social Work and Research* at 10 years of age and counting: an idea whose time had come. *Research on Social Work Practice*, 15, 3–7.

Padgett, D.K. (1998). *Qualitative methods in social work research*. Thousand Oaks, CA: Sage.

Pawson, R. (2006). *Evidence-based policy: a realist perspective*. London: Sage.

Pawson, R. and Tilley, N. (1997). *Realistic evaluation*. London: Sage.

Pawson, R., Greenhalgh, T., Harvey, G. and Walshe, K. (2005). Realist review: a new method of systematic review designed for complex policy interventions. *Journal of Health Services Research Policy*, 10 (Supplement 1), 21–34.

Pawson, R., Greenhalgh, T., Harvey, G. and Walshe, K. (2004). *Realist synthesis: an introduction*. RMP Methods Paper 2/2004, ESRC Research Methods Programme, University of Manchester.

Payne, M. (2002). Social work theories and reflective practice. In Adams, R., Dominelli, L. and Payne, M. (eds). *Social work: themes, issues and critical debates* (2nd edn). Basingstoke: Palgrave. 123–138.

Pease, B. and Fook, J. (1999). *Transforming social work practice*. St Leonards: Allen and Unwin.

Peile, C. (1988). Research paradigms in social work: from stalemate to creative synthesis. *Social Service Review*, 62(1), 1–19.

Penka, C.A. and Kirk, S.A. (1991). Practitioner involvement in clinical evaluation. *Social Work*, 36(6), 513–518.

Pincus, A. and Minahan, A. (1973). *Social work practice: model and method*. Itasca, Illinois: F.E. Peacock Publishers.

Plano Clark, V.L. and Creswell, J.W. (2007). *The mixed methods reader*. London: Sage.

Plath, D. (2008). Evidence-based practice. In Gray, M. and Webb, S.A. (eds). *Social work theories and methods*. London: Sage. 172–183.

Plath, D. (2006) Evidence-based practice: current issues and future directions. *Australian Social Work*, 59(1), 56–72.

Plath, D., English, B., Connors, L. and Beveridge, A. (1999). Evaluating the outcomes of intensive critical thinking instruction for social work students. *Social Work Education*, 18(2), 207–217.

Platt, D. (2007a). Advice to care home operators on strategies for successful outcomes of social care inspections. *Journal of Care Services Management*, 1(1), 12–18.

Platt, D. (2007b). *The status of social care: a review 2007*. London: Department of Health, HMSO.

Platt, D. (2002). *Guidance on the single assessment process for older people*. London: Centre for Policy on Ageing.

Platt, D. (1996). *Then ... Now ... Onwards*. Birmingham, UK: British Association of Social Workers.

Platt, D. (1992). Contracting and agreements with the voluntary sector: an SSD view. In Allen, I. (ed.). *Purchasing and providing social services in the 1990s*. London: Policy Studies Institute.

Proctor, E.K. (2007). Implementing evidence-based practice in social work education: principles, strategies, and partnerships. *Research on Social Work Practice*, 17(5), 583–591.

Proctor, E.K. and Rosen, A. (2008). From knowledge production to implementation: research challenges and imperatives. *Research on Social Work Practice*, 18(4), 285–291.

Putnam, H. (1999). *Problems with the observational/theoretical distinction*. Oxford: Oxford University Press.

Rapp-Paglicci, L. (2007). Book review of Roberts and Yeager 2004 and 2006, *Research on Social Work Practice*, 17, 427.

Reid, W.J. (2001). The role of science in social work: the perennial debate. *Journal of Social Work*, 1(3), 273–293.

Reid, W.J. (1997). Evaluating the dodo's verdict: do all interventions have equivalent outcomes? *Social Work Research*, 21(7), 5–15.

Reid, W.J. (1994). The empirical clinical practice movement. *Social Service Review*, June, 165–184.

Reid, W.J. (1980). Research strategies for improving individualized services. In Fanshel, D. (ed.). *Future of social work research*. Washington, DC: National Association of Social Workers.

Research in Practice (2008). *Think research: using research evidence to inform service development for vulnerable groups*. Social Inclusion Unit, Cabinet Office, HM Government, UK.

Richmond, M. (1917). *Social diagnosis*. New York: Russell Sage Foundation.

Risan, L. (1997). Artificial life: a technoscience leaving modernity? An anthropology of subjects and objects. Retrieved 23 October 2008. http://www.anthrobase.com/Txt/R/Risan_L_05.htm

Ritzer, G. (2004). *Encyclopedia of Social Theory*. London: Sage Publications.

Roberts, R.W. and Nee, R.H. (eds). (1970). *Theories of social casework*. Chicago: University of Chicago Press.

Roberts, A.R. and Yeager, K.R. (eds). (2006). *Foundations of evidence-based social work practice*. New York: Oxford University Press.

Roberts, A.R. and Yeager, K.R. (eds). (2004). *Evidence-based practice manual: research and outcome measures in health and human services*. New York: Oxford University Press.

Rodwell, M.K. (1998). *Social work constructivist research*. New York: Garland Publishing, Inc.

Rogers, E.M. (1995). *Diffusion of innovations* (4th edn). New York: Free Press.

Rohlin, M. and Mileman, P.A. (2000). Decision analysis in dentistry: the last 30 years. *Journal of Dentistry*, 28(7), 453–468.

Ronen, T. (2004) Evidence-based practice in Israel. In Thyer, B.A. and Kazi, M.A.F. (eds). (2004). *International perspectives on evidence-based practice in social work*. Birmingham, UK: Venture Press. 113–132.

Ronen, T. (1994). Cognitive behavioural social work with children. *British Journal of Social Work*, 24, 273–285.

Roseborough, D. (2006). Psychodynamic psychotherapy: an effectiveness study. *Research on Social Work Practice*, 16, 166–175.

Rosen, A. (2003). Evidence-based social work practice: challenges and promise. *Social Work Research*, 27(4), 197–207.

Rosen, A. (1994). Knowledge use in direct practice. *Social Service Review*, 68, 561–577.

Rosen, A. and Proctor, E. (2003). *Developing practice guidelines for social work intervention*. New York: Columbia University Press.

Rosenblatt, A. and Waldvogel, D. (eds). (1983). *Clinical social work handbook*. San Francisco: Jossey Bass.

Rostila, I. and Piirainen, K. (2004). Evidence-based practice in Finland. In Thyer, B.A. and Kazi, M.A.F. (eds). (2004). *International perspectives on evidence-based practice in social work*. Birmingham, UK: Venture Press. 197–213.

Ross, L. (1977). The intuitive psychologist ad his shortcomings. In Berkowitz, L. (ed). *Advances in Experimental Social Psychology*. Academic Press, New York.

Rubin, A. (2008). *Practitioner's guide to using research for evidence-based practice*. Hoboken, New Jersey: John Wiley and Sons.

Rubin, A. (2007a). *Research on Social Work Practice*, 334–347.

Rubin, A. (2007b). Improving the teaching of evidence-based practice: introduction to the Special Issue. *Research on Social Work Practice*, 541–547.

Rubin, A. (2007c). Epilogue: the Austin initiative. *Research on Social Work Practice*, 17, 630–631.

Rubin, A. and Babbie, E. (2008). *Research methods for social work* (6th edn). Belmont, CA: Brookes/Cole.

Rubin, A. and Parrish, D. (2007a). Views of evidence-based practice among faculty in Master of Social Work programs: a national study. *Research on Social Work Practice*, 17(1), 110–122.

Rubin, A. and Parrish, D. (2007b). Problematic phrases in the conclusions of published outcome studies: implications for evidence-based practice. *Research on Social Work Practice*, 17(3), 334–347.

Ruckdeschel, R.A. (1985). Qualitative research as a perspective. *Social Work Research and Abstracts*, 21(2), 17–21.

Ruckdeschel, R.A. and Farris, B.E. (1981). Assessing practice: a critical look at the single-case design. *Social Casework*, 62(7), 413–419.

Sackett, D.L., Rosenberg, W., Gray, J.A.M., Haynes, R.B. and Richardson, W.S. (1996). Evidence-based medicine; what it is and what it isn't. *British Medical Journal* (312), 71–72. http://cebm.jr2.ox.ac.uk/ebmisisnt.html

Sackett, D.L., Straus, S.E., Richardson, W.S., Rosenberg, W. and Haynes, R.B. (2000). *Evidence-based medicine: how to practice and teach EBM* (2nd edn). New York: Churchill Livingstone.

Sackett, D.L., Straus, S.E., Richardson, W.S., Rosenberg, W. and Haynes, R.B. (1997). *Evidence-based medicine: how to practice and teach EBM*. New York: Churchill Livingstone.

Sandell, R., Blomberg, J., Lazar, A., Carlsson, J., Broberg, J. and Schubert, J. (2000). Varieties of outcome among patients in psychoanalysis and long-term psychotherapy: a review of findings in the Stockholm Outcome of Psychoanalysis and Psychotherapy Project (STOPP). *International Journal of Psychoanalysis*, 56, 343–359.

Sanderson, I. (2002). Making sense of 'what works': evidence based policy making as instrumental rationality? *Public Policy and Administration*, 17, 61–75.

Schwartz, A. (1983). Behavioral principles and approaches. In Rosenblatt, A. and Waldvogel, D. (eds). *Clinical social work handbook*. San Francisco: Jossey Bass.

Schwarz, N. (1998). Accessible content and accessibility experiences: the interplay of declarative and experiential information in judgment. *Personality and Social Psychology Review*, 2, 87–99.

Scott, D. (2002). Adding meaning to measurement: the value of qualitative methods in practice research. *British Journal of Social Work*, 32, 923–930.

Scott-Findlay, S. and Pollock, C. (2004) Evidence, research, knowledge: a call for conceptual clarity, *Worldviews on Evidence-Based Nursing*, 1(2), 92–97.

Scourfield, P. (2006). 'What matters is what works'? How discourses of modernization have both silenced and limited debate on domiciliary care for older people. *Critical Social Policy*, 26, 5–30.

Sebba, J. (1999) 'Setting priorities for systematic reviews'. Paper presented at the Campbell Collaboration meeting, University College, London, 15–16 July. Available online at: http://www.ucl.ac.uk/spp/download/publications/SPP-FIN.pdf

Shadish, W. and Myers, D. (2004). *Campbell Collaboration research design policy brief*. Campbell Collaboration. Retrieved 22 September 2008. http://camp.ostfold.net/artman2/uploads/1/Research_Design_Policy_Brief.pdf

Shaw, I. (2003). Cutting edge issues in social work research. *British Journal of Social Work*, 33, 107–120.

Shaw, I. (1999). Evidence for practice. In Shaw, I. and Lishman, J. (eds). *Evaluation and social work practice*. London: Sage. 14–40.

Shaw, I. and Shaw, A. (1997). Game plans, buzzes and sheer luck: doing well in social work. *Social Work Research*, 21(2), 69–79.

Shek, D.T.L., Tang, V.M.Y. and Han, X.Y. (2005) Evaluation of evaluation studies using qualitative research methods in the social work literature (1990–2003): evidence that constitutes a wake-up call. *Research on Social Work Practice*, 15(3), 180–194.

Sheldon, B. (2001). The validity of evidence-based practice: a reply to Stephen Webb. *British Journal of Social Work*, 31(6), 801–809.

Sheldon, B. (1986). Social work effectiveness experiments: review and implications. *British Journal of Social Work*, 6, 223–242.

Sheldon, B. and Chilvers, R. (2000). *Evidence-based social care: a study of prospects and problems*. Lyme Regis: Russell House Publishing.

Sheldon, B. and Macdonald, G. (1999). *Research and practice in social care: mind the gap*. Exeter: Centre for Evidence-Based Social Services.

Sheldon, B., Chilvers, R., Ellis, A., Moseley, A. and Tierney, S. (2004). An empirical study of the obstacles to evidence-based practice. In Bilson, A. (ed.). *Evidence-based practice in social work*. London: Whiting & Birch Publishers.

Sheppard, M. (2006). *Social work and social exclusion*. Aldershot, Hants: Ashgate.

Sherman, E. and Reid, W.J. (1994). *Qualitative research in social work*. New York:

Columbia University Press. 251–264.

Sherman, L.W. (2003). Misleading evidence and evidence-led policy: making social science more experimental. *Annals of the American Academy of Political and Social Sciences*, 589, 6–19.

Shibano, M. (2007). In search of evidence of a child's best interests: bridging research and practice in social work. In Furukawa, A. (ed.). *Frontiers of social research: Japan and beyond.* Melbourne: Trans Pacific Press. Chapter 13.

Shibano, M. (2004). Behavioral family treatment in Japan: design and development of a parent training program. In Briggs, H.E. and Rzepnicki, T.L. (eds). *Using evidence in social work practice: behavioral perspectives.* Illinois: Lyceum Books Inc. 210–230.

Shlonsky, A. (in press). Teaching evidence-based practice in social work. In Roberts, A. (ed.). *Social Worker's Desk Reference* (2nd edn). New York: Oxford University Press.

Singleton, V. and Michael, M. (1993). Actor-networks and ambivalence: general practitioners in the UK Cervical Screening Programme. *Social Studies of Science*, 23, 227–264.

Smalley, R. (1970). General characteristics of the functional approach: a brief statement of the origins of this approach. In Roberts, R.W. and Nee, R.H. (eds). *Theories of social casework.* Chicago: University of Chicago Press.

Smedslund, G., Dalsbo, T.K., Steiro, A.K., Winsvold, A. and Clench-Aas, J. (2007). Cognitive behavioural therapy for men who physically abuse their female partner. *Cochrane Database of Systematic Reviews*, Issue 3, Art. No.: CD006048. DOI:10.1002/14651858. CD006048.pub2.

Smith, D. (ed.). (2004). *Social work and evidence-based practice.* London: Jessica Kingsley Publishers.

Smith, D. (1987). The limits of positivism in social work research. *British Journal of Social Work*, 17(4), 401–416.

Smith, L. Tuhiwai. (1999). *Decolonizing methodologies: research and indigenous peoples.* New York: St Martin's Press.

Social Care Institute of Excellence (SCIE) (2007). Boardpapers, July, London. Retrieved 23 September 2008. http://www.scie.org.uk/publications/boardpapers/july02.asp

Soydan, H. (2008). Applying randomized controlled trials and systematic reviews in social work research. *Research on Social Work Practice*, 18, 311–318.

Soydan, H. (2007). Improving the teaching of evidence-based practice: challenges and priorities. *Research on Social Work Practice*, 17(5), 612–618.

Sparks, C. (2007). Reality TV: the Big Brother phenomenon. *International Socialism*, 114. Retrieved 5 November 2008. http://www.isj.org.uk/index.php4?id=314&issue=114

Spiro, S. (2007). Review of *Foundations of Evidence Based Social Work Practice* edited by Albert R. Roberts and Kenneth Yeager. *British Journal of Social Work*, 37, 367–369.

Spratt, T. and Houston, S. (1999). Developing critical social work in theory and in practice: child protection and communicative reason. *Child and Family Social Work*, 4, 315–324.

Staller, K.M. (2006). Railroads, runaways, and researchers: returning evidence rhetoric to its practice base. *Qualitative Inquiry*, 12(3), 503–522.

Stanfill, C. and Waltz, D. (1986). Toward memory-based reasoning. *Communications of the ACM*, 29(12), 1213–1228.

Statens Offentliga Utredningar (SOU) (2008). *Evidensbaserad praktik inom socialtjänsten: Till nytta för brukaren* (Evidence-based practice: for the service user's benefit). Stockholm: Statens Offentliga Utredningar.

Steketee, G. (1999). Yes, but cautiously. *Research on Social Work Practice*, 9(3), 343–346.

Stradling, J.R. and Davies, D.M. (1997). The unacceptable face of evidence-based medicine. *Journal of Evaluation in Clinical Practice*, 3(2), 99–103.

Strauss, S.E., Richardson, W.S., Galsziou, P. and Haynes, R.B. (2005). *Evidence-based medicine: how to practice and teach EBM* (3rd edn). New York: Elsevier.

Stronach, I. and Hustler, D. (2001). Old whine in new battles. *British Educational Research Journal*, 27(5), 523–525.

Sundell, K., Brännström, L., Larsson, U. and Marklund, K. (2008). *På väg mot evidensbaserad praktik: 834 kommunala enhetschefer om evidensbaserad praktik och användning av evidensbaserade metoder inom socialtjänstens verksamhetsområden*. (Toward evidence-based practice: 834 municipal social work agency directors about evidence-based practice and utilization of evidence-based interventions in the activity fields of social work). (Working Paper, 28 August 2008). Stockholm: IMS.

Surry, D.W. (1997). *Diffusion theory and instructional technology*. Available online at: http://intro.base.org/docs/diffusion/

Taylor, S.E. (1981). The interface of cognitive and social psychology. In Harvey, J.H. (ed.). *Cognition, social behaviour and environment*. Philadelphia: Lawrence Erlbaum.

Teddlie, C. and Tashakkori, A. (2008). *Foundations of mixed method research*. London: Sage.

Tenner, E. (1996). *Why things bite back: technology and the revenge of unintended consequences*. New York: Alfred A. Knopf.

Timmermans, S. (2008). Professions and their work: do market shelters protect professional interests? *Work and Occupations*, 35,164–188.

Thomas, E.J. (1967). *The socio-behavioral approach and applications to social work*. New York: CSWE.

Thyer, B.A. (2008a). Intervention with adults. In Rowe, W. and Rapp-Paglicci, L. (eds). *Comprehensive handbook of social work and social welfare: Volume 3 – Social work practice*. New York: Wiley. 326–347.

Thyer, B.A. (2008b). The quest for evidence-based practice? We are all positivists! *Research on Social Work Practice*, 18(4), 339–345.

Thyer, B.A. (2007). Social work education and clinical learning: towards evidence-based practice? *Clinical Social Work Journal*, 35, 25–32.

Thyer, B.A. (2006). What is evidence-based practice? In Roberts, A. and Yeager, K. (eds). *Foundations of evidence-based social work practice*. Oxford University Press: Oxford. 35–46.

Thyer, B.A. (2002). Evidence-based practice and clinical social work. *Evidence Based Mental Health*, 5, 6–7.

Thyer, B.A. (1991). Guidelines for evaluating outcome studies on social work practice. *Research on Social Work Practice*, 1(1), 76–91.

Thyer, B.A. (1989). First principles of practice research. *British Journal of Social Work*, 19, 309–323.

Thyer, B.A. and Kazi, M.A.F. (eds). (2004). *International perspectives on evidence-based practice in social work*. Birmingham, UK: Venture Press.

Timmermans, S. and Berg, M. (2003). *The gold standard: the challenge of evidence-based medicine and standardisation in health care*. Philadephia: Temple University Press.

Trinder, L. (2000). A critical appraisal of evidence-based practice. In Trinder, L. and S. Reynolds (eds). *Evidence-based practice: a critical appraisal*. Oxford: Blackwell Science.

Trinder, L. and Reynolds, S. (eds). (2000). *Evidence-based practice: a critical appraisal*. Oxford: Blackwell Science.

Tyson, K. (1995). *New foundations for scientific social and behavioral research: the heuristic paradigm*. Needham Heights, MA: Allyn and Bacon.

Upshur, R.E.G., Van Den Kerkhof, E.G. and Goel, V. (2001). Meaning and measurement: an inclusive model of evidence in health care. *Journal of Evaluation in Clinical Practice*, 7(2), 91–99.

US Department of Health and Human Services. (2006). *The road ahead: research partnerships to transform services.* A report by the National Advisory Mental Health Council's Services Research and Clinical Epidemiology Workgroup. Available online at: http://www.nimh.nih.gov/about/advisory-boards-and-groups/namhc/reports/road-ahead.pdf

van de Luitgaarden, G.M.J. (2007). Evidence-based practice in social work: lessons from judgment and decision-making theory. *British Journal of Social Work*, Advance Access published on 30 November 2007. DOI: doi:10.1093/bjsw/bcm117.

Van Zyl, M.A. (2004), Evidence-based practice in South Africa. In Thyer, B.A. and Kazi, M.A.F. (eds). (2004). *International perspectives on evidence-based practice in social work.* Birmingham, UK: Venture Press. 133–148.

Varela, F.J. (1999). *Ethical know-how: action, wisdom and cognition.* Stanford, CA: Stanford University Press.

Wakefield, J. and Kirk, S.A. (1996). Unscientific thinking about scientific practice: evaluating the scientist–practitioner model. *Social Work Research*, 20, 83–95.

Walsham, G. and Sahay, S. (1999). GIS for district-level administration in India: problems and opportunities. *MIS Quarterly*, 23(1), 39–65.

Walter, I., Nutley, S., Percy-Smith, J., McNeish, D. and Frost, S. (2004). Improving the use of research in social care practice. *SCIE Knowledge Review 7.* London: Social Care Institute of Excellence. Retrieved 23 September 2008. http://www.scie.org.uk/publications/knowledgereviews/kr07.aspe

Wambach, K.G., Haynes, D.T. and White, B.W. (1999). Practice guidelines: rapprochement or estrangement between social work practitioners and researchers. *Research on Social Work Practice*, 9, 322–330.

Wampold, B.E. (2001). *The great psychotherapy debate: models, methods and findings.* Mahwah, NJ: Lawrence Erlbaum, Publishers.

Warburton, B. and Black, M. (2002). Evaluating processes for evidence-based health care in the National Health Service. *British Journal of Clinical Governance*, 7(3), 158–164.

Watson, M. (2003). Using the internet for evidence-based practice. In Harlow, E. and Webb, S.A. (eds). *Information and communication technologies in the welfare services.* London: Jessica Kingsley Publishers.

Webb, S.A. (2008). Evidence-based social work: the actuarial re-casting of social work. *The Indian Journal of Social Work*, 45(3), 135–148.

Webb, S.A. (2006). *Social work in a risk society: social and political perspectives.* London: Palgrave Macmillan.

Webb, S.A. (2002). Evidence-based practice and decision analysis in social work: an implementation model. *Journal of Social Work*, 2(1), 45–63.

Webb, S.A. (2001). Some considerations on the validity of evidence-based practice in social work. *British Journal of Social Work*, 31, 57–79.

Webb, S.A. and Harlow, E. (eds). (2003). *Information and communication technologies in the welfare services.* Jessica Kingsley: London.

Weick, A. (1987). Reconceptualising the philosophical perspective of social work. *Social Service Review*, 61(2), 218–230.

Weissman, M.M., Verdeli, H., Gameroff, M., Bledsoe, S.E., Betts, K., Mufson, L., *et al.* (2006). A national survey of psychotherapy training programs in psychiatry, psychology, and social work. *Archives of General Psychiatry*, 63, 925–934.

Weissman, M.M. and Sanderson, W.C. (2001). Promises and problems in modern psycho-therapy: the need for increased training in evidence-based treatments. In Hager, M. (ed.). *Modern psychiatry: challenges in educating health professionals to meet new needs.* New York: Josiah Macy Jr. Foundation. 132–165.

White, B.W. (ed.) (2008). *Comprehensive handbook of social work and social welfare: the profession of social work, Volume 1.* New Jersey: John Wiley and Sons, Inc.

White, S. (2008). Discourse analysis and reflexivity. In Gray, M. and Webb, S.A. (eds). *Social work theories and methods.* London: Sage, 161–171.

Williams, F., Popay, J. and Oakley, A. (eds). (1999). *Welfare research: a critical review.* London: Routledge.

Witkin, S.L. (1996). If empirical practice is the answer, then what is the question? *Social Work Research*, 20(2), 69–75.

Witkin, S.L. (1992). Should empirically-based practice be taught in BSW and MSW programs? No! *Journal of Social Work Education*, 28, 265–269.

Witkin, S.L. (1991). Empirical clinical practice: a critical analysis. *Social Work*, 36(2), 158–163.

Witkin, S.L. and Gottschalk, S. (1988). Alternative criteria for theory evaluation. *Social Service Review*, 62(2), 211–224.

Witkin, S.L. and Harrison, W.D. (2001). Whose evidence and for what purpose? *Social Work*, 46: 293–296.

Wolpe, J. (1969). *The practice of behavior therapy.* New York: Pergamon.

Woolf, S.H. *et al.* (1999). Potential benefits, limitations, and harms of clinical guidelines. *British Medical Journal*, 318, 527–530.

Woolf, S.H., DiGuiseppi, C.G., Atkins, D., and Kamerow, D.B. (1996). Developing evidence-based clinical practice guidelines: lessons learned by the US Preventive Services Task Force. *Annual Review of Public Health*, 17, 511–538.

Yin King Lee, L. (2003). Evidence-based practice in Hong Kong: issues and implications in its establishment. *Journal of Clinical Nursing*, 12, 618–624.

Zlotnik, J. (2007). Evidence-based practice and social work education: a view from Washington. *Research on Social Work Practice*, 17(5), 625–629.

Zlotnik, J., DePanfilis, D., Daining, C. and Lane, M.M. (2005). *Factors influencing retention of child welfare staff: a systematic review of research.* Washington, DC: Institute for the Advancement of Social Work Research.

Index

Entries in **bold** denote text in figures and tables.

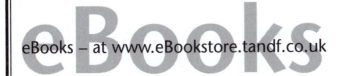

eBooks – at www.eBookstore.tandf.co.uk

A library at your fingertips!

eBooks are electronic versions of printed books. You can store them on your PC/laptop or browse them online.

They have advantages for anyone needing rapid access to a wide variety of published, copyright information.

eBooks can help your research by enabling you to bookmark chapters, annotate text and use instant searches to find specific words or phrases. Several eBook files would fit on even a small laptop or PDA.

NEW: Save money by eSubscribing: cheap, online access to any eBook for as long as you need it.

Annual subscription packages

We now offer special low-cost bulk subscriptions to packages of eBooks in certain subject areas. These are available to libraries or to individuals.

For more information please contact webmaster.ebooks@tandf.co.uk

We're continually developing the eBook concept, so keep up to date by visiting the website.

www.eBookstore.tandf.co.uk